Disability and Disadvantage

DAVID LOCKER

Disability and Disadvantage

THE CONSEQUENCES OF
CHRONIC ILLNESS

TAVISTOCK PUBLICATIONS
LONDON AND NEW YORK

First published in 1983 by
Tavistock Publications Ltd
11 New Fetter Lane, London EC4P 4EE

Published in the USA by
Tavistock Publications
in association with Methuen, Inc.
733 Third Avenue, New York, NY 10017

Photoset by
Nene Phototypesetters Ltd, Northampton
Printed in Great Britain by
J. W. Arrowsmith Ltd, Bristol.

British Library Cataloguing in Publication Data

Locker, David
Disability and disadvantage.
1. Rheumatoid arthritis
2. Handicapped – Great Britain –
    Social conditions
I. Title
362.1'96722'0941   RC933
ISBN 0–422–78740–X

Library of Congress Cataloging in Publication Data

Locker, David.
Disability and disadvantage.
(Social science paperbacks)
Bibliography: p.
Includes index.
1. Rheumatoid arthritis – Addresses, essays, lectures.
2. Rheumatoid arthritis – Patients – Great Britain – Economic
conditions – Addresses, essays, lectures.   3. Rheumatoid
arthritis – Patients – Great Britain – Social conditions –
Addresses, essays, lectures.   4. Chronically ill – Great
Britain – Economic conditions – Addresses, essays, lectures.
I. Title.   II. Series.   [DNLM: 1. Chronic disease.
2. Handicapped. 3. Arthritis, Rheumatoid.   WE 346 L815d]
RC933.L58 1983   305'.90816   83–4971
ISBN 0–422–78740–X (pbk.)

Contents

For R.N.H.

Acknowledgements

So many people helped with the writing of this book that it is difficult to know where to begin. The most significant contribution was made by the twenty-four people who provided the data on which the book is based. They willingly gave their time and energy and tolerated physical discomfort so that their experience of living with disability could be documented during lengthy interviews. In some ways it is a pity they must remain anonymous. Many colleagues in the Department of Community Medicine, St Thomas' Hospital Medical School assisted in innumerable ways, particularly those comprising the Physically Handicapped Study Team. Prominent among them were: Professor W. W. Holland, Donald Patrick, Steven Green, Geoff Horton, Ellie Scrivens, and Myfanwy Morgan. Thanks are due to Queenie Parrish of the British Rheumatism and Arthritis Association and those Rehabilitation Officers who helped in the search for the people interviewed in the study and also to Joan Camus who typed the manuscript and provided much needed editorial advice. For their continuing encouragement and support I am grateful to Richard Howard, Geoff Posner, Peter Lancaster, Dick Stabbins, Alice Smith, Jill Woolford, Simon Pullen, Ruth Watson, Jill Evans, Judith McCann, Paula and Michael Grey, Hugh Davidson, Françoise Picard, Maureen Gaudet, Paul and Annie Flower, and David Morgan.

Introduction

There is no doubt that disabled people are a severely disadvantaged minority within British society. Numerous studies have shown that in terms of income, employment, housing, and access to facilities in the community, they are markedly worse off than their non-disabled counterparts. Despite almost a century of provision for disabled people, many are still excluded from full participation in community life. In some respects they are a hidden minority, confined in their own homes or, in some instances, within institutions either in the community or remote from centres of population. Consequently, there is only limited public awareness of their existence and probably less of their needs.

This book is concerned with the disadvantage and deprivation experienced by a small group of individuals severely disabled by one disease, rheumatoid arthritis. It is not so much concerned with the proportions and percentages of the disabled population who do not have jobs, adequate incomes, or homes adapted to their needs but with detailed description of the disadvantage some disabled people experience in their everyday lives. It examines the problems they encounter from day to day and their own efforts at solving, or at least containing, them. It is concerned with the consequences of chronic illness and the never-ending struggle of coping they involve, both for the individual with a limiting disorder and members of his or her family. A great deal of attention is given to the resources the group of people had available to them and the strategies they employed to manage problems and provide for a more satisfactory daily life.

Two main themes are pursued in the book. The first is that disabled people disadvantaged because chronic illness and the limitations in activity it produces result in a loss of personal, material, and social resources, and the resources that remain are almost wholly consumed in the effort of coping with the illness and its effects. The second is that the resources disabled persons can muster and the problem-solving strategies they are able to construct are factors which intervene between impairment, disability, and disadvantage. These themes are illustrated by data drawn from lengthy and detailed interviews with twenty-four people limited by rheumatoid arthritis. Each of these people was interviewed twice in his or her own home using a semi-structured approach which allowed for a description of a wide range of problems and experiences. The major part of the book consists of extracts taken directly from those interviews.

Chapter 1 offers the briefest of summaries of major themes in the sociological literature on chronic illness and disability and concentrates on those works from which the theoretical ideas on which the book is based were drawn. These ideas are largely to do with meaning, disadvantage, and everyday life. These pages can probably be omitted by the general reader more interested in disabled people than sociological theory. The remainder of the chapter describes the data collection procedures and offers a brief description of the characteristics of the people who agreed to participate in the study. Chapter 2 looks at the problems created by the disease itself, its major symptoms, their effects and how they are managed in the course of daily life. It describes the disruption created by pain and uncertainty and the way in which chronic illness makes the everyday world a world fraught with danger. Chapter 3 is concerned with problematic aspects of medical care, ranging from the difficulties the people experienced in their encounters with health professionals to the distressing effects of therapeutic interventions.

Chapter 4 discusses the practical problems of everyday life, focusing on ambulation, mobility, self care, and household management. It describes the way in which mundane matters loom large in the context of disability and tries to convey something of the struggle disabled people face in simply getting through the day. Chapter 5 examines work and income and describes some of the consequences of unemployment and poverty. It examines the way in which the organization of work excludes people disabled by rheumatoid arthritis and looks at their experience of discrimination in the labour market. Also considered are their attempts to maximize incomes and their strategies for managing with much reduced financial resources. Chapter 6 offers an analysis of problems in the sphere of social relationships and family life. Data is presented to illustrate the problems of legitimacy, stigma, and dependency and the extent to which a chronic illness impinged on their performance of marital and parental roles. Chapter 7 describes the cognitive and interactional problems that emerged during contacts with the welfare agencies charged with improving the lot of disabled people and ends with a brief case study of a crisis in one of the families contacted to demonstrate the way in which formal and informal help may disable as well as enable. As with the chapter on medical care, the successes of the welfare system are largely ignored in order to concentrate on the failures. This seemed justified in a work that is predominantly concerned with the problems these twenty-four people faced and the way in which the illness and their attempts to cope with it created a great deal of distress.

The work is intended to say something about the nature of the disadvantage which stems from one chronic limiting disorder and to convey something of the experience of being a disabled person. While the analysis does have theoretical and policy implications which are discussed in the concluding chapter, it was not intended to give rise to recipes for transforming the health and social care of disabled people. This study was one of a group of five conducted by a research team of social scientists, medical statisticians, and epidemiologists, and the task of identifying health promoting interventions and more effective social policy options for the physically disabled population is one best left for the team as a whole in the light of the data from the accumulated studies. Collectively, they offer a prevalence estimate of disability in the community, an epidemiology of the course of impairment and disability, a scaling study designed to provide British weightings for a comprehensive measure of disability originally constructed in the USA, a study of the priorities of disabled people, and this study of handicap or the disadvantage consequent upon chronic illness. These studies have been completed or are currently nearing completion and are described in Patrick *et al.* (1981; 1982). They were financed by the Department of Health and Social Security and conducted within the Health Services Research Unit and Department of Community Medicine, St Thomas' Hospital Medical School, London.

1 An approach to chronic illness and disability

Studies of chronic illness and disability drawing on the social sciences have been many and varied and fall into one of four main categories. The first consists of studies, primarily epidemiological in character, which have been concerned with the definition and measurement of chronic illness and disability, their prevalence in defined communities and the identification of the causes of the major disabling conditions. Since the late 1960s a number of government sponsored and independent research efforts have documented the numbers and needs of the disabled population in Britain (Townsend 1967; Jefferys *et al.* 1969; Harris 1971; Patrick *et al.* 1981a; 1981b; 1982). Secondly, there are studies falling within the area of rehabilitation which have attempted to identify the social and psychological factors influencing behavioural responses to disease and injury (Litman 1962; Rossillo and Fogel 1970; Hyman 1975; Susset *et al.* 1979; Fross *et al.* 1980; Smith and Midanik 1979). Thirdly, there are studies of disabled people, their problems, and the contribution of welfare provision (Blaxter 1976; Burton 1975; Bayley 1973; Wilkin 1979), and finally, there are attempts to provide a specifically theoretical understanding of chronic illness and disability by the application of a variety of sociological perspectives (Goffman 1963; Davis 1963; Freidson 1965).

A major problem encountered in some, but by no means all, of this literature is an inconsistent use of terminology. While administrative definitions of disability are often clear cut (Blaxter 1976), the use of terms like impairment, disability, and handicap has been unsatisfactory with little regard for the nature of the events to which they refer. Townsend (1967) has gone so far as to claim that imprecision in the use of terminology and the conceptual confusion it embodies was one reason for the lack of systematic information on chronic illness and its consequences. Wood (1975; 1980) has resolved this problem by devising the now familiar taxonomy which has been adopted for international use by the World Health Organisation. His concepts of impairment, disability, and handicap refer to related though radically different areas of human experience. Accordingly, impairment is defined as any disturbance in body structures or processes which are present at birth or arise from disease or injury. Disabilities were originally defined as limitations in the functions customarily expected of the body or its parts *or* restrictions in activity consequent upon impairment. More recently, this definition has been modified so that functional limitations are classified as impairments in order to make the boundary between impairment and disability more clear cut. Handicap is the social disadvantage originating in impairment and disability because the individual does not or cannot conform to the expectations and taken-for-granted assumptions of the society or social groups to which he or she belongs: any loss or abnormality of body structure and function may have an impact on life chances and limit the attainment of material and social rewards. This concept of handicap is a useful one because it clearly differentiates the social consequences of disease from disease itself and provides one point of departure for a sociology of chronic illness and disability. According to Wood, handicap is a social construct, dependent upon meanings and values, and is the prime area of sociological concern. Wood's contribution goes further, however, in that he not only defines three major areas of human experience but links them in the manner shown in *Figure 1*.

Figure 1   Wood's representation of the links between impairment, disability, and handicap

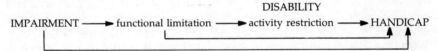

As this representation suggests, handicap may be a consequence of a linear progression along the full sequence of events. It may also be a direct consequence of aspects of an impairment which are neither functionally limiting nor disabling; for example, a facial disfigurement which creates embarrassment and disadvantage in social interaction. Handicap may also be a direct consequence of the functional limitations associated with a given impairment even though there is no disability which intervenes. Wood quotes the example of a child with coeliac disease who is able to live a normal life in terms of activity but may be handicapped by an inability to share a common diet.

In the context of this discussion it is probably of more importance to note that the relationships between impairment, disability, and handicap are not direct but are mediated by a number of as yet ill-defined factors. The disability that may result from a given impairment is not a direct function of anatomical loss or degree of functional limitation but is influenced by self-conception, social support, definition of the illness, and many other variables. A neat example is to be found in the recent work of Fross *et al.* (1980) who studied children with asthma. Groups, comparable in terms of the severity of their asthma, as indexed by measures of pulmonary function, differed significantly in terms of reported incapacitation and interference with daily life. A key factor was the child's response to the illness. Those with high levels of fear and panic were far more disabled than those with low levels. Similarly, the relationship between disability and handicap is not direct; handicap is historically and culturally variable (Hanks and Hanks 1948; Freidson 1965). Since handicap is dependent on social meanings and social values, it is also socially relative. Consequently, a given attribute or incapacity may result in disadvantage in one group or society but not another, or it may be handicapping at one point in time but not another. The so-called mentally handicapped are disadvantaged in modern industrial societies because social organization takes for granted a certain level of cognitive ability and because verbal intelligence and intellectual skills are highly valued and highly rewarded (Dexter 1964). In other societies, or at other historical periods, intellectual impairment and social incompetence may not be similarly consequential.

Evidence for the deprivation experienced by disabled people in Britain is to be found in a number of studies. Sainsbury (1970) examined the housing, employment, and income characteristics of those registered in the general classes of physically disabled in three areas and found that, relative to the general population, they were severely disadvantaged in all three. McLean and Jefferys (1974) showed that considerable changes in social status occurred following the onset of disability in a group of men suffering spinal injury; these men experienced significant downward occupational and economic drift. In a study based on a national sample, Harris (1971) found very high rates of unemployment among disabled people; of those severely disabled only 30 per cent were working, and of those appreciably disabled only 50 per cent had jobs. A national survey of household standards of living reaffirmed the differences in income between the disabled and non-disabled (Townsend 1979). The proportion of people with appreciable or severe disabilities living on incomes on the margins of the State's standard of poverty was three times that of the non-disabled. Similar patterns have been found in a more recent study of an inner city community (West 1982; Somerville 1982). Even when employed, disabled people are more likely to be low paid and less likely to have assets in the form of savings, personal possessions, and consumer durables (Townsend 1979).

While these studies are valuable as evidence of disadvantage and indispensable to the political process of securing additional resources for the disabled population, they are not without limitations. Firstly, disadvantage is more pervasive than these studies would suggest; disabled people are worse off than the non-disabled who share their low standards of living, poor housing, and lack of occupational opportunities. As a number of studies on the families of handicapped children have shown, a significant aspect of being or caring for a disabled person is the 'daily grind' it entails; the never-ending and unrewarded hard work involved in coping with a chronic condition and the numerous mundane practical problems to which it gives rise. This daily grind is a constant drain on already limited resources. One study estimated that the mothers of severely disabled children spend 10 hours per week dealing with incontinence alone (Townsend and Heng 1981). Secondly, these studies are also limited because they focus on outcomes rather than the processes which produce those outcomes.

Theoretical approaches

As Bury (1982) has recently suggested, medical sociologists interested in chronic illness and disability have drawn on two contrasting theoretical traditions. The first derives from Parsons' analysis of the sick role and his concept of illness as deviance (Parsons 1951). On the one hand this has given rise to a rather sterile debate about the relevance of the expectations defining the sick role for understanding chronic illness (Kassebaum and Baumann 1960) and an equally sterile depiction of disability as deviance (Freidson 1965). As Bury goes on to note, a more promising elaboration of Parsons' work is that which draws on his notion of health as adaptation (Gallagher 1976; Gerhardt 1979), a theme developed at length by Haber and Smith (1971) in an earlier and neglected paper. While the idea of adaptation might be limited in that it tends to imply stability, when most chronic disabling disorders are not stable and unchanging, it does have a certain continuity with some of the work derived from the second tradition, that of symbolic interactionism. Not unexpectedly, this work has largely been concerned with meaning and identity. These themes are prominent in the early studies of Goffman (1961) and Roth (1963) whose analyses of the way in which illness is created and shaped by social definition and institutional management gave rise to the concept of the illness career and echoed the claims of the labelling theorists in their approach to deviance. Deviance and mental illness were not attributes of individuals but properties conferred on them by others, the social pressures involved leading to the adoption of a social role and the stabilization of relevant patterns of behaviour (Becker 1963; Scheff 1966). The idea of adaptation is, however, closer to the concerns of a second body of research produced within this overall perspective, that of the management of problematic aspects of chronic illness and disability. The classic studies of Goffman (1963) and Davis (1963) concentrated on the problems experienced by the chronically sick and disabled in their encounters with normals. Within this work, and its elaboration by others (Edgerton 1967; Birenbaum 1970), is a detailed specification of the way in which routine social interaction is managed by the discredited and discreditable in order to cope with stigma and the threat to their public identity. More recently published studies have extended this approach and developed an understanding of the strategies employed to deal with symptoms, medical crises, and therapeutic regimens (Strauss 1975; Reif 1973; Fagerhaugh 1973) and the uncertainty created by an unstable, fluctuating disorder (Wiener 1975). These studies have begun the work of documenting in detail the problems created by chronic illness and disability and their consequences in everyday life. In a sense, adapting to a long-term disabling illness involves reconstructing everyday life in order to avoid, minimize, or otherwise manage its disruptive effects.

Disability, disadvantage, and everyday life

As Blaxter (1976) has suggested, the meaning of chronic illness and disability is to be found in the problems it creates both for the sufferer and his or her family. In the short term the onset of such an illness constitutes a critical incident, disrupts taken-for-granted assumptions about the past and future and calls for some kind of explanation which will give meaning to this unexpected event (Bury 1982). In the longer term it results in a reduction in physical resources so that the mundane practical matters of everyday life can no longer be taken for granted but become problems that need to be solved. While these problems may not differ radically in kind from those experienced by non-disabled people and the acutely ill (Shearer 1981: 29; Strauss 1975: 9), they do differ in frequency, intensity, and duration. For some disabled people, daily life is no longer one of freely competing for social and material rewards since necessary resources such as time, energy, and money are absorbed by the sheer effort of coping with symptoms and getting through the day. Disabled people are handicapped to the extent that the pool of resources available to them is greatly reduced and what remains must be employed in order to accomplish the mundane. Accordingly, an inability to get out of bed or get to the toilet without help is as much a part of the disadvantage experienced by the disabled as unemployment and social isolation. To the extent that it impedes their access to and participation in community life, difficulty with the ordinary practical matters of everyday life constitutes and creates disadvantage.

The extent to which functional limitations and activity restrictions constitute a problem, or are otherwise handicapping, is not only variable historically and culturally but is also somewhat dependent upon more immediate contexts; their meaning is not the same across different social and environmental settings. To take a simple example, the loss of one finger may have different consequences for a professional musician and a manual labourer in terms of occupational opportunities. Similarly, an inability to climb stairs is of more significance for someone living on the fifth floor of a block of flats without a lift than it is for someone living in a ground floor flat. The meaning of a given functional limitation or activity restriction is also likely to be influenced by the resources and problem solving strategies an individual commands and constructs since these will have a bearing on the extent to which the problematic aspects of attributes and activities consequent upon disease and impairment can be successfully managed. A sensitivity to the significance of context allows the study of the problems faced by chronic sufferers to be placed within wider theoretical concerns; the maldistribution of resources in society affects the ability of individuals from different socio-economic groups to maintain a satisfactory existence in the face of a long-term disabling disorder (Bury 1982).

Initially, however, this study is concerned with the meaning of impairment and disability in terms of the disadvantage experienced by individuals and families following the onset of a chronic limiting disorder. This is pursued empirically by an analysis of the nature and dynamics of problems disabled people encounter in everyday life, the resources available to them to compensate for loss of faculty and the strategies they employ to reduce the impact of such loss on life chances. In this way it continues the work of Strauss and colleagues who have sought to understand the daily experiences of the chronically sick person by focusing on key problems, basic strategies, and changes in the organization of family life. To the extent that the data on which the work is based allows for an analysis of careers, some attempt is made to examine the ways in which the meaning of impairment and disability is transformed over time as a result of changes in social and personal circumstances. By way of an introduction, some preliminary comments can be made concerning types of problems, types of resources, and types of strategies.

The problems disabled people encounter can be broadly categorized in the following way. Medical problems arise directly from the disease or impairment and take the form of symptoms which need to be controlled in various ways; it includes the problems which arise from medical intervention and professionally prescribed regimens. Cognitive problems consist of the difficulties involved in attempting to make sense of the onset, course, and future of the disorder and also problems in understanding the workings of the medical and welfare agencies which offer treatment and social support. The practical problems of everyday life consist of difficulties in mobility, self-care, and household management. Interactional problems include difficulties encountered in social interaction, social relationships, and family life and encompass the major problems of stigma and social isolation. Occupational problems arise in the attempt to acquire or maintain a meaningful role within the workforce and in the consequences of unemployment, and economic problems arise from the loss of income or financial independence and the practical and symbolic effects of poverty.

The resources chronically sick and disabled persons command can also be classified according to type; they may be physical, cognitive, material, or social. They reflect life chances prior to the onset of illness and disability and may be important determinants of life chances following onset. Medical and social services can be considered to be resources on which disabled people may draw and like the others may be acquired or lost during the course of the person's career. These resources figure significantly in the strategies that are used to cope with problems since coping mechanisms invariably draw on knowledge, time, personal help, or material effects like aids or appliances. Such strategies must be brought to bear on all the difficulties the chronically sick and disabled people encounter and are changed or modified as the resources on which they depend become available or are finally consumed. In fact, the daily life of those with a limiting condition can be characterized as one in which goods and services are constantly and carefully allocated and reallocated in order to gain the maximum from whatever is available. Some idea of the range of strategies necessary to cope with such an illness can be gained from the work of Reif (1973) and Wiener (1975). The former has described the preventive, protective, and corrective strategies used by people with ulcerative colitis to cope with the problem of personal pollution, and the latter has identified the social strategies of covering up, keeping up, and pacing by means of which people with rheumatoid arthritis attempt to normalize an existence dominated by pain, immobility, and reduced energy. While the published papers of Reif and Wiener have provided a number of important insights, they are largely concerned with the way in which problems arising directly from the disorder itself may be contained. The following chapters attempt to take a wider view and offer a detailed description of a broad range of difficulties imposed on a group of people by chronic illness and disability. Throughout, resources and strategies are viewed as variables which intervene between disability and handicap.

The respondents and the data

The approach briefly outlined above is elaborated in the following chapters using data derived from semi-structured interviews with twenty-four people severely disabled by rheumatoid arthritis, whose disability was not of recent origin, and who lived within the borders of an inner London borough. Eleven of the individuals were located as a result of an epidemiological survey designed to produce a prevalence estimate of disability within the borough (Patrick *et al.* 1981a), nine were contacted via the case loads of the rehabilitation officers employed by the local Social Services Department, and the remainder were contacted through the local branch of the Rheumatism and Arthritis Association. Since no attempt was made to identify and randomly sample from the total population of sufferers within the borough, this strategy had the advantage of producing a group of individuals who differed widely in their social and personal characteristics. This is useful in a study which proceeds by means of detailed case histories. People with rheumatoid arthritis were chosen because it is a relatively common disorder,[1] can be very disabling at an early age, is a progressive, fluctuating condition which requires a high degree of self-management, is of unknown aetiology with available treatments being palliative, empirical, and often unsuccessful, and can be but is not necessarily visibly deforming. In short, it epitomizes many of the issues of interest in chronic illness and highlights the complex relationship between disability and disadvantage.

Each of the participants was interviewed twice in his or her own home, and both interviews were tape recorded. The first interview was based on a common schedule of topic headings and probes and was designed to cover as wide a range of their experiences as possible. The second interview was based on a similar schedule modified to take account of what each had said at the first interview but focused on changes in impairment, disability, and social and personal circumstances. The interviews were conducted one year apart. Some questions were designed to collect factual information about the respondents' condition and their circumstances, although most were designed to stimulate them to give lengthy accounts of their experiences as disabled people. The quantity of data this produced frequently meant that each interview required two and sometimes three visits to be completed. In five cases the spouse was present during the interview and in one case a daughter. Since these were the people providing the bulk of care and support, their contribution to the interview was welcomed even though it meant that some topics, for example, family relationships, had to be approached more carefully. Their accounts of their caring role have been used in order to underline the point that disability in one member can encompass the family as a whole.

Sixteen of the individuals were female and eight male and in age ranged from 24 to 64 years, ten being in their fifties. Twelve were married, six had never married, four were widowed, and two divorced or separated. Nine lived alone, nine with one other person, and six with two or more relatives. All gave a diagnosis of rheumatoid arthritis, and three had additional chronic disorders. Mrs K had been diagnosed as having multiple sclerosis, and because her speech was affected, her husband assisted in the conduct of the interviews; Mr H had a chest condition which produced severe breathlessness, and Mrs G had the most complex medical history; she was blind, diabetic and, as well as arthritis, was subject to another painful condition she referred to as myositis or polyneuritis.[2] Although the onset of impairment and disability was difficult to date, many of those interviewed had been significantly affected for a number of years. At one end of the scale were Mr M and Mr I who had been disabled and unemployed for two and three years respectively, and at the other, Mrs T, who was 53 when first seen and who had been disabled since childhood. The majority had been chronically ill, if not limited, for ten years or more. The youngest, Mrs D, was diagnosed at the age of fourteen, and by the age of 24 was very disabled and visibly deformed by the disease. At the start of the study, Mr H was bed-bound, Mrs W, Mrs T, and Mrs R confined to wheelchairs, and apart from seven people who could go out alone, the remainder were housebound or dependent on help to get out of the house. In terms of broad categories, half of the respondents were very severely or severely disabled, needing help with some aspect of personal care; the other half were moderately disabled and while self-care activities were always difficult they could be performed without help. Three of the respondents lived with disabled spouses.

Eleven of the respondents were middle class and thirteen working class. Because the majority were women and because many seemed to occupy the grey area between the two major groupings, the classification procedure was at times rather arbitrary. At the time of the first interview, only one of the respondents, Miss L, was working although Mrs A was employed but on extended sick leave from work, and Mr M was hoping to go back to his old job. Some of the others wanted to work but were far from clear as to how they might re-enter the work force, while some had given up all idea of ever working again.

Some idea of the diversity among the respondents can be gained from a few brief descriptions. Mrs J lived with a disabled husband and five daughters aged between 14 and 21 in a run-down Victorian terraced house badly affected by damp. She had lived in that area of the city all her life and was the centre of a close knit and extended family network. Her main problems were the poor housing conditions in which she lived and the effort of managing a household while chronically ill. Mr H was virtually bed-ridden and lived with his wife in a modern block of flats purpose-built for the severely disabled. Having owned their own business and their own home, the H's were relatively financially secure but almost totally isolated socially with little in the way of family and no friendship network; this had disintegrated as he became increasingly disabled. Mrs G lived alone and was struggling to manage in her flat in the face of a number of chronic disorders and increasing levels of pain. She had three sons and one daughter who lived on the outskirts of London, but having been ill for most of their childhood refused to call on them for help. Her main problem was in trying to find some way of controlling pain so that she could become mobile again and return to her job as a teacher of the blind. She was very critical of her medical care and as hope

Table 1 *Personal characteristics of respondents*

name	age	years since onset (estimated)	family composition	household composition	last occupation	mobility status
Mrs A	56	16	Married No children	Husband, 51	Senior secretary	Independently mobile
Miss B	64	12	Single	Lives alone	Laundry worker	Housebound
Mr C	42	24	Single	Lives alone	Manual labourer	Limited outdoor mobility
Mrs D	24	10	Separated No children	Cohabitee, 37	Typist	Housebound
Mr E	59	15	Married 1 son	Wife, 57	Lorry driver	Independently mobile
Mr F	44	4	Married 1 daughter 1 son	Wife, 44 daughter, 17 son, 12	Skilled manual labourer	Limited outdoor mobility
Mrs G	55	25	Widowed 1 daughter 3 sons	Lives alone	Teacher	Housebound
Mr H	59	22	Married No children	Wife, 56	Manager	Bed/wheelchair bound
Mr I	41	3	Married 2 daughters 1 son	Wife, 38 daughters, 13 and 11 son, 14	Caretaker	Housebound
Mrs J	39	12	Married 5 daughters 1 son	Husband, 65 daughters, 20, 19, 18, 16, 14	Housewife	Independently mobile
Mrs K	54	7	Married 4 daughters 3 sons	Husband, 60	Shop assistant	Needs help outdoors

Name	Age		Marital status	Household	Occupation	Mobility
Miss L	49	12	Single	Sister, 44 nephew, 11	Clerk (employed)	Independently mobile
Mr M	48	2	Single	Lives alone	Assistant manager	Independently mobile
Mrs N	53	6	Married 2 daughters	Husband, 51	Clerk	Independently mobile
Mrs O	58	20	Married 2 daughters	Husband, 60	Housewife	Limited outdoor mobility
Mr P	63	19	Single	Lives alone	Lift attendant	Limited outdoor mobility
Mrs Q	62	22	Widowed All children deceased	Lives alone	Housekeeper	Housebound
Mrs R	62	38	Divorced 3 daughters	Daughter, 24 son in law, 30	Clerk	Wheelchair bound
Mr S	55	32	Married 1 daughter 2 sons	Wife, 46 son, 16	Print machine operator	Limited outdoor mobility
Mrs T	53	45	Married No children	Husband, 54	Office manager	Wheelchair bound
Mrs V	64	27	Widowed 3 sons	Lives alone	Waitress	Housebound
Mrs W	59	29	Married No children	Husband, 56	Clerk	Wheelchair bound
Mrs X	61	31	Widowed 3 daughters 1 son	Lives alone	Clerk	Limited outdoor mobility
Miss Z	36	7	Single	Lives alone	Ward orderly	Independently mobile

of improvement faded began to consider the possibility of residential care. Mr I lived with his wife and three teenage children in a small, decaying flat in a block built at the turn of the century. The I's main problems were poor housing, isolation, and poverty, and the struggle to improve their lot in the face of a system of welfare provision which seemed to them to be complex, remote, and uncaring. Miss L lived on the top floor of a house occupied by her sister and nephew. She had a clerical job with the Civil Service and valued the independence that an income of her own made possible. Her life was organized in a manner which she hoped would maximize her chances of remaining in work so that she could avoid having to be dependent upon others. The characteristics of all twenty-four respondents are summarized in *Table 1* (pages 10–11).

While diverse the individuals making up the group shared a number of characteristics. They all had rheumatoid arthritis, they were all disabled, and all had reorganized their daily existence in order to cope with the disease and its effects. Although their problems were common there was a measure of variation in the degree to which they were experienced by individual respondents. The most severely disabled in the group were often the most significantly affected and frequently provided the most vivid illustrations of the consequences of chronic illness. This was not always the case, however. At times the less severely disabled people experienced problems more acutely and this was sometimes a function of the stage of the career of the illness, sometimes related to current levels of pain, and sometimes to their individual responses to the difficulties they faced. Like many disabled people, the fundamental need of the people in this study was for social acceptance, integration, and unimpeded access to the opportunities that life in a complex industrial society makes possible (Walker 1981). In the following chapters some of their problems and needs are described in detail.

The tape recorded interviews were transcribed in full so that the data consists of the respondents' accounts of their disorder and its treatment, their disabilities and their consequences in everyday life, and their encounters with the medical and welfare bureaucracies to which they turned for help and support. In the following pages numerous and sometimes lengthy extracts from the transcripts of the interviews are presented.[3] Throughout, preference has been given to what the respondents themselves had to say. There are two reasons for this. Firstly, it means the analysis can be judged against the data from which it was derived; secondly, there is no doubt that the problems of disabled people are better described in their own words rather than my secondary elaborations of them. The accounts were sometimes punctuated to make them readable, but other than this they are presented as said.

The main aim of the book is to offer a detailed description of the everyday disadvantage experienced by a small group of disabled people.

Even though a small group of individuals, it was sometimes possible to observe patterns across the group, and these are described particularly where they reflect the patterns reported by others who have used larger and random samples. Some effort has been made to avoid covering in detail areas that have already been amply covered in the enormous literature on the disabled population. This was not always possible or desirable since it would have meant leaving gaps in what was intended to be a broad view of their circumstances and struggles. It is hoped that such overlap will verify and elaborate and not prove too tedious for the reader already familiar with the literature and disabled people.

Notes

1. It has been estimated that 10 per cent of persons have some form of arthritis and approximately one third of these will have rheumatoid arthritis. In men the prevalence rate of rheumatoid arthritis is 1.7 per cent and is substantially higher in women at 4.6 per cent (Kitkay 1977). Osteoarthritis is even more common with rates being two and a half times higher than for the rheumatoid form. This latter disease affects men and women in equal proportions. Diseases of the bones and joints are the commonest causes of disability and of those so afflicted approaching 75 per cent will have arthritis of one type or another. While less common than osteoarthritis rheumatoid arthritis is more likely to lead to severe disability (Knight and Warren 1978).
2. Throughout the book the respondents are identified by letter only.
3. In the extracts where Int. appears this refers to the interviewer, i.e. the author.

2 *Living with rheumatoid arthritis*

Many of the problems experienced by people limited by rheumatoid arthritis are common to all who are appreciably disabled in some way. Unemployment, an inadequate income, social isolation, and a sense of being a burden on others are reported by a high proportion of the disabled population irrespective of the specific disorder which produces their disability. Other problems, however, are not common to all with a chronic disorder since they originate in the nature of the particular impairment and the way it manifests itself in symptoms. For example, a person with ulcerative colitis is faced with the problem of personal pollution (Reif 1973), the person with emphysema has to contend with breathlessness and an inadequate oxygen supply (Fagerhaugh 1973), and the cardiac patient must cope with the fear of sudden death. Similarly, rheumatoid arthritis has a number of characteristics which produce specific problems for those so afflicted. In fact, the early stages of the disabled person's career may consist entirely of a process of learning to cope with and adapt to the symptoms of the disease itself rather than the wider social consequences that follow appreciable disability. In this respect, the biological realities that constitute disease, though mediated by individual and societal responses, have an important impact on an individual's daily life and life chances. Consequently, this chapter is concerned with the practical and cognitive problems posed by the symptomatic character of rheumatoid arthritis and the way these are managed in the course of everyday life.

Rheumatoid arthritis is an incurable disease of unknown aetiology which produces swelling and inflammation of the supporting tissues of joints throughout the body.[1] It is more common in women than men and though it does occur in childhood, onset is typically during the thirties or forties (Hughes 1979). In the majority of cases the onset is insidious and symptoms may be present for months or even years before it is finally diagnosed or gives rise to appreciable disability. Onset is usually signalled by pain in one joint, often in the upper or lower extremities, and this pain may disappear and reappear several times before it spreads to other joints. In a few cases the velocity of the illness is more rapid, and severe involvement of many joints develops soon after the initial symptoms appear with the person becoming severely disabled over a very short period of time. Here the impact of the disease on the person and the family can be quite catastrophic, producing a sudden and dramatic decline in their social and material circumstances.

The main symptom of rheumatoid arthritis is pain in one or, more usually, several joints throughout the body. While the level of pain may fluctuate both in the short and long term, it is virtually always present and often inescapable; life may be organized so as to minimize the level of pain experienced but it can rarely be avoided altogether. As Miss L commented in talking about her pain, 'Everything you do means pain. I sometimes think I wish I could have just one day without pain.' In the later stages, when the disease becomes 'burnt out', levels of pain subside and may disappear from some if not all of the affected joints. This may take fifteen or twenty years or more if it happens at all. The life of a person with rheumatoid arthritis is, then, overwhelmingly a life of pain; waking life is dominated by pain and structured by the strategies adopted to avoid or minimize it.

During acute phases of the disease or on what many of the respondents described as 'bad days', the pain was severe and unremitting and at times totally overwhelming. At the second interview Mrs T was in the middle of an acute attack and talked at length about her pain.

> *Mrs T:* At this particular instance it's quite bad, my knees, my shoulder, my neck . . . this particular pain and its level I've had for five or six days now and it's not altered at all, it's not got worse, it's not got better and it's not spread but it's just gone on and on and, God, I am *so* tired.

Even when the pain is not that severe, it is still devastating in its effects, predominantly because it is always there.

> *Mrs T:* Whenever anybody has asked me to explain the pain my description has not been on the pain itself but what it does to you; the loss of energy because all your energy is concentrated on trying to cope with it, the tiredness and the weariness and the monotony of the continual, not necessarily violent, but the continual nagging pain that's there when eventually you go to sleep. You wake up and the first conscious thing that is there you think 'O God', and you know the chances are it's going to be with you the whole of the day.

While the pain experienced on 'bad days' may be severe, it is tolerable simply because there is a foreseeable end. The next day, or at least the day after, will be a 'good day'; the pain will subside and may even be absent while the person is sitting or lying down. What makes the pain of acute attacks particularly distressing is that there is no foreseeable end and no possibility of relief. Mr F's only acute attack lasted for almost two years, and during that time he tried any number of remedies in the hope of easing the pain.

> *Mr F:* This was the thing that used to get me, was no matter what you done, even the pain killers I had, they done no good and, believe me, I took some tablets. I'd try anything, you know, just to get rid of the pain, but no matter what I took it didn't make any difference. I think this was what was really getting on my nerves, the fact that I couldn't get rid of the pain. I tried everything, the lot; ice cubes, boiling water, sun-ray lamps, the lot.

Others described how they continually attempted to find a body position that would give them some degree of comfort and moved from chair to bed and back again or, like Mr M, tried lying on the floor. While in bed they tried lying on their right side, then their left, and then their back. Contrary to his doctor's instructions, Mr F placed pillows under his knees and tried sleeping with his right leg out of the bed in order to avoid the weight of the covers and on particularly bad nights abandoned the bed altogether in favour of the settee. Some bought or were given special chairs and mattresses, and some made repeated visits to the doctor in the hope that one of the drugs currently available would prove to offer a degree of relief. When these manoeuvres turned out to be ineffective, when lying, sitting, standing, and moving about were all equally painful, the individual often reached the edge of despair. As Mrs W commented, 'You just don't know what to do with yourself.'

With rheumatoid arthritis these acute phases or flare-ups are followed by periods of remission when levels of pain subside, mobility improves, and the symptoms of the disease are not so totally overwhelming. The phases when the disease is not so active may last for many years, and over time pain became accepted as a normal feature of everyday existence, so normal that its absence and not its presence gives rise to comment. Mr S said 'If I don't wake up in pain I think there's something wrong with me.' The respondents also came to accept a given level of pain as normal, and this provided a marker by which day-to-day fluctuations were judged and dosages of drugs varied. When Mr I tried to reduce the volume of steroids he was taking, the result was pain and swelling of the joints in his legs and neck. Over the following two days he doubled the dosage until he was back to normal, 'Well, I say back to normal, back to what I am now.' Many of the people in this study described how they had 'learned to live with pain', and they were sometimes unsure as to whether the pain had subsided or whether they were now so used to pain that it no longer had that great an impact on them. The process of normalizing pain was, however, highlighted when called into question by more active phases of the disease.

Mrs R: My pain has increased about twofold over the last couple of years and I'm going through a kind of transitional period where I have to . . . with a rheumatic complaint there is always a basic sort of pain. It hurts when I move but there's always been a basic pain level which over the years I have quite truthfully been able to accept as discomfort rather than pain. You say that's normal, so you don't call that pain, you just call it discomfort. Well, my discomfort over the last two years has risen twofold at least, so I'm in the transitional period of endeavouring to accept that as the norm. I'm not able to at the moment because a steady pain is extremely tiring and I've not yet accepted that as normality. I am finding it extremely tiring.

As well as giving rise to pain, rheumatoid arthritis damages the tissues in the joints so that they become stiff and limited in their range of movement. Initially, joints may be kept immobile in the effort to reduce pain; subsequently, they become deformed and misshapen or may lock so that movement becomes impossible. Atrophy of the muscles controlling the joints leads to a loss of strength, dexterity, and manual skills so that the capacity to lift, carry, and manipulate objects is substantially reduced. While mobility produces additional pain, attempting to contain pain by immobility results in a stiffening of the joints so that subsequent movement is difficult and even more painful. Many of the respondents balanced these contradictory demands by alternating rest and movement. They all avoided sitting for longer than an hour and would walk around the room periodically in order to loosen the joints. When this was not possible or when they allowed themselves to sit for too long, they often had to be lifted out of the chair and spend time and effort in getting going again. After Mr I had spent the evening watching television, he was always stiff and stood for ten mintues before he even attempted to move.

A second and highly problematic characteristic of rheumatoid arthritis is the variable and unpredictable pattern it routinely follows (Wiener 1975). This total absence of predictability adds to the burden of managing the day-to-day manifestations of the disease. Not only does it add to the cognitive problem of making sense of the disease and its course, it also adds to the practical problem of minimizing and containing its symptoms. The occurrence of flare-ups and their duration is always uncertain; no one can predict when they will happen or for how long they will last. Consequently, during a period of remission there is always the fear that tomorrow may bring another flare-up and weeks or months of additional suffering. Though the disease is progressive, its end point is also uncertain. Individuals affected may expect to get worse but do not know with any certainty whether they will end up bed-bound and totally dependent or whether the disease will go into spontaneous remission before they reach that stage. Uncertainty is also present on a day-to-day level. The only certainty is that there will be pain; how much, which joints will be affected and how mobile they will be is never known in advance. Consequently, rheumatoid arthritis is a disease which requires continuous monitoring and self-management since little can be taken for granted.

The day-to-day variation in the symptoms of rheumatoid arthritis was characterized by all of the respondents as one of 'good days' and 'bad days' during which levels of pain and disability fluctuated wildly. Mr M's description was typical.

> *Mr M:* Well, with this complaint it's just one of those things you get good days and bad days. Some days you're all. . . . Well, you're never all right but the pain is not so great, it's up and down like a yo-yo. Some days you feel ruddy marvellous and could jump over the moon, other days you're fit for nothing.

This variability would be less problematic if it was not complicated by uncertainty; as it was, most were reduced to living from day to day and just had to wait and see. Some, like Mrs O, took a pain reading early in the morning and planned the day accordingly; by the time she had got out of bed, got to the bathroom and finished washing, 'I'm as good as I'm going to be during the day'. The highly erratic character of the disease often forestalled such attempts to attain a measure of predictability since the location of the pain and its intensity often varied throughout the course of the day. Mrs W said 'I wake up with the pain here and it goes somewhere else till you've got all the pain under the sun', and Mrs J said 'I can get up in the morning and feel on top of the world but by twelve o'clock I'll be stuck in a chair. It's just the way arthritis goes.'

For all the respondents, pain was not only an unpleasant experience in itself but also a source of limitation; actual or anticipated pain was as, if not more, disabling than the damage the disease did to the joints and their supporting structures. Limbs capable of mobility were rendered immobile by pain or the fear of pain so that controlling this pain became a concern overriding all others. For example, Mrs G had been blind for a number of years but had travelled across London by bus to a centre where she taught other blind people to read braille. She had only become housebound when the pain of her arthritis and associated complaints became continuous and severe.

> *Mrs G:* If I can get the pain under control then of course the mobility becomes easier. Say a paraplegic, although their legs are useless they're not in pain. You see, what you do then is slide yourself in a car and chuck your legs in after and that's it, but if that's so painful that you can't even contemplate the idea that's a bugbear pain. If I can get the pain under control we're laughing. You see, blind people are mobile, your eyesight or lack of it doesn't keep you at home.

While pain and the fear of pain are sources of inactivity, they are compounded by one of the other major effects of the disease, a loss of energy. The metabolic effects of rheumatoid arthritis reduce reserves of energy which are further reduced by the necessity of coping with continuous pain. Consequently, activity, however minimal, requires physical and psychological effort. Mrs T described the problem in the following way.

> *Mrs T:* What makes the biggest impact on people is when I talk about the lack of energy and the fact that for me to lean across the table and pick that up which is something they would do without thinking about it and without really any consciousness causes me pain and takes a tremendous effort to do it and I don't *want* to do it because nobody if they've got pain wants to make it worse. I have to expend six or seven times the energy to even open and close a door and I haven't got that much energy in the first place.

In the face of pain and lack of energy, activity has to be reduced to a bare minimum. Even so, some activities are unavoidable, particularly so for the person who lives alone who is forced to cope with basic essentials like toileting and eating. These relatively minor tasks require a period of preparation before the arthritic person is ready to attempt them.

> *Mrs G:* At the moment I'm doing practically nothing because I can't. I'm having literally to screw up courage in the morning to get up to go into the bathroom. I have to . . . everytime I want to do something I have to steel myself first to do it.

When the physical and psychological effort is not forthcoming, then the person simply gives up. Even ordinary activities like making a cup of tea or turning on the television may not be done since the necessity to overcome pain, stiff and weak joints, and the malaise and lowness that accompany the disease is just too much. In fact, the psychological effort sometimes proved to be the greater barrier to activity. As Mrs A said 'It's necessary to whip up enthusiasm to do things rather than it being automatic and this is not the sort of person I was.' At the time of the first interview, Mr F only ever left the house to go for physiotherapy and heat treatment at the hospital but would often miss appointments rather than have to cope with the problem of getting there.

> *Mr F:* I just haven't got the stamina to stand up to it, you know, if you're in pain and that and, er, I just don't bother to go. I've just got that attitude, you could say it's a state of mind really, but it's, erm, it really takes a big effort, even normally it takes a big effort to go down to the bus stop. It's only up the road but I just won't walk up, you know. It isn't that I don't want to it's, er, I can never get into the frame of mind to push myself far enough. It's just the thought of that walk.

Sometimes if he was comfortable in bed, Mr F would lie there all day rather than struggle to rally the psychological resources necessary to get him going. Even so, staying in bed involved a certain cost: 'I was used to getting up early. With my job it was nothing to travel around the country so staying in bed did depress me but I didn't have the courage or the energy to bother getting out.' Looking back on this period he said, 'I just couldn't have cared less about anything and anybody. I didn't have the will to do anything.'

Depression and frustration are not symptoms of rheumatoid arthritis but consequences of the disease and its disabling effects. Both were very common among this group of people and so prominent a part of everyday existence that some believed that depression at least was a manifestation of the disorder itself rather than a part of their response to it. Both depression and frustration were a product of incapacity and arose when planned activities had to be abandoned because of pain, when ordinary activities were attempted and found to be out of reach, and when jobs had to be left when only half completed; that is, whenever their identity as damaged and disabled persons was reaffirmed in the course of everyday activity. For some, incapacity and the frustration to which it gave rise were often harder to bear than the pain:

> *Mrs J:* It drives me mad it really does, I could bang my head against the wall. I can't bear to be incapacitated. I want to do what I want to do and not what me hands want me to do and that is what gets me.

Although a consequence rather than a symptom, depression was very distressing and had to be managed in much the same way as the other manifestations of the disorder.

> *Mrs W:* Depression is one of the worst things. I don't know if it goes with this complaint, I think it must do. Depression is the worst thing absolutely. Some days it's dreadful. You sit there thinking 'I don't think I'll get up, I'll just sit here.' And there's all this terrible pain going up your arms. But I do have terrible days sometimes. You have days when you get very depressed, it's a very depressing complaint. You've got all this pain and you think 'God, I wish I knew what to do with myself,' and then you hear somebody's killed themselves and you think 'It's a good idea really.' And then you come to your senses and think it's damn stupid. When I get depressed I think, 'There's people worse off than I am,' and I try to think of all the people I know at my club who are ten times worse than me and I think how lucky I am. And I think 'Put some music on, that'll do it, that'll cheer me up.' But I do get very depressing days, very painful days when you go to pick something up or cut something and there's pain.

The problematic character of the pain

The rheumatoid arthritic person's experience of pain is surrounded by uncertainty. The pain varies in its intensity, duration and location in the various joints of the body. It is also unpredictable, and individuals can never accurately forecast how they are going to be. These characteristics of variability and unpredictability make the pain itself more difficult to manage and exacerbate the disruptive effect of pain on social and personal life. For example, because pain may be present in one joint one day and another the next, the kinds of everyday activities they are able to undertake are constantly changing, and the nature of the difficulty they have in doing a given task also changes. Shaving may be difficult one day because of limited movement in the shoulders and difficult the next because the hands cannot get a grip on a razor. Consequently, coping on a day-to-day level requires the use of a wide repertoire of strategies in order to meet these shifting eventualities. In addition, it may mean that methods of pain control are not always successful. Mrs T found that analgesics gave some relief on days when the level of pain was average but none whatsoever when the pain was severe. Similarly, because they never knew when the pain was going to be bad or when a prolonged flare-up was going to occur, forward planning was impossible. As Mr I said: 'It's hard to say until you wake up in the morning you don't know what you are going to wake up to. You couldn't say to anybody, "Don't come tomorrow I'm going to be bad."' Mrs R managed this uncertainty by living from day to day so that forward planning was unnecessary.

> *Mrs R:* This is another thing with this complaint you can't make arrangements, you've got to do things when you can. I never plan ahead, I can't, there's no good in planning ahead 'cus I just don't know how I'm going to be from one day to the other.

Other respondents attempted to cope with this uncertainty somewhat differently. Mrs X had an understanding with her family and friends that any arrangements they made were subject to cancellation at short notice, and her daughters were quite used to her telephoning to ask that they not visit because she was in too much pain. Another illustration of the way the problem may be collectively managed is evident in the case of Mrs N and her family. Mrs N and her husband always used to accompany their daughters and their families on an annual holiday to Spain. When Mrs N's arthritis deteriorated, 'it had to stop, we could never book up anywhere 'cus I never knew how it was going to be.' Consequently, the entire family pooled their resources and bought a caravan which was kept on the coast and available for Mrs N to use whenever she felt well: 'It's better to have this knowing I can't book up to go away.'

As well as being unable to predict when levels of pain will increase or flare-ups occur, the person with rheumatoid arthritis often cannot explain why this should happen. Even the day-to-day variation of the symptoms may be something of a mystery.

> *Mrs A:* I often feel this when I'm talking to my consultant, it doesn't show a precise pattern does it. I mean sometimes people say 'Does the weather affect you?' Well it does but not always. The pouring rain and the bitter cold sometimes does. On a day like today when it's warm and humid it can be absolute agony yet another time when it's bitterly cold I'm going around merrily. I just don't know, it doesn't follow a precise pattern at all and this is what fools you, you wake up in the morning and you just have to wait and see how you are going to be that day.

Mr M also found it difficult to specify what it was that caused the pain to get worse: 'That's a thing that mystifies me, some people say it's the weather, but you can never pin it down to one thing.' Where such increases in pain cannot be explained and where no cause can be identified, the individual is left mystified and confused. Mrs G said 'Some days I seem almost free and then I get a week like this, I don't understand why it isn't constant.' Such confusion adds to the distress of living with pain and means that protective strategies for avoiding events which lead to pain are sometimes difficult to construct. Consequently, some effort was invested in the attempt to discover what exacerbated pain, either by monitoring day-to-day experience or seeking expert advice.

> *Mr M:* I've asked the doctor several questions you know. Why is it I get good days and bad days? Why is it I can go reasonably well along and another day I come to a dead stop? Well, he reckons I'm overdoing it, he said I should try and keep to the same pace all the time.

Such advice allowed them to perceive some pattern to their experience and meant explanations could be constructed which tied the pain to some prior activity.

> *Mr M:* Today is a bad day, I'm in quite a lot of pain actually, but there again I went out yesterday and so I'm suffering for it today.

Such connections suggest their own remedy; pain can sometimes be controlled by resting and taking it easy. This is not the end of the matter, however, for the individual is then faced with the difficult choice of living a limited life and keeping pain levels down or attempting to do more with the risk that he or she will suffer additional pain. As Wiener (1975) has discussed, the person with rheumatoid arthritis has to balance the physiological imperative and the activity imperative in order to avoid unacceptable levels of pain or an unacceptable degree of invalidity. Mrs A found this choice so problematic that she sought guidance from her consultant.

Mrs A: He said 'The only patients I've had with your complaint who have improved have done so after they've led a quieter life.' He said very firmly that I should take a good two hours rest every day. Well I don't, but I do sit down after lunch for a while and I think rest is a good thing. We were talking about this when I went to see him last month and I said 'You know, there are days when I don't do very much and I end up at the end of the day with a guilty conscience and there are days when I do considerably more and I end up with a great deal of pain but no guilty conscience.' And he said 'Well, there's no contest, have the guilty conscience.'

Because the constraints imposed by the physiological imperative were often judged to be unacceptable, the activity imperative sometimes won out and pain became the price that had to be paid for indulging in activity. Mrs A followed her consultant's advice only selectively and sometimes undertook activities she knew would result in pain: 'Quite often I think "Well, I know this is going to have the effect on me but I'll do it anyway." ' Like Mrs A, Mrs T thought pain a less undesirable option than withdrawing from the general run of everyday life and refused to avoid the stressful situations she believed led to physical discomfort.

Mrs T: If I do see that it's wise for me to keep out of a particular situation I don't necessarily avoid it because that to me is an avoidance of one's responsibility in life. Just because one has a chronic complaint it doesn't mean that it should be used as an excuse to opt out and to wrap oneself up away from life.

Because their doctors continually advised them to rest or because experience had taught them that activity means pain, some of the respondents did try as far as possible to organize their lives in such a manner that long periods of time were spent resting. Miss L's main concern was keeping well enough to remain at work and retain her financial independence. Since most of her energy was consumed by work, she kept her social activities to a minimum, always went to bed early and rested as much as she could. She found that spending one day entirely alone when she need do very little seemed to do her a lot of good, and in order to inconvenience others as little as possible she used her annual leave in this way.

Miss L: I like to do it without thinking 'What do people think downstairs?' At weekends people are around and I don't like to withdraw from it so sometimes I take days from my holiday. Last year I took most of my holiday as one day off a week so I could be totally by myself. It means I don't get a proper holiday but it is beneficial.

In cases such as these, keeping well involves considerable costs. The

effort not only consumes material resources such as time but also results in a less varied and satisfying existence. As Miss L commented later in the interview: 'It is annoying because it means you've got to live life like a cabbage.'

Other explanations of variations in the intensity of pain were equally problematic in terms of their implications for pain control. For example, many of the respondents mentioned physical and emotional stress as a cause of additional pain and tried as far as possible to avoid situations where this was likely. This was not always easy, as Mrs A said, 'in this day and age how can you possibly manage that', since stressful circumstances were not always of their own making. While Miss L tried not to do too much lifting and carrying at work, there came a point where she had to do her share of physical labour so as not to jeopardize her relationships with colleagues. Tension and pain could result from minor matters like the irritation of having to wait three-quarters of an hour for a bus or from more threatening events like rifts in family relationships. The former cannot be avoided while the latter may call for major changes in life circumstances. Miss L used to live with her sister and brother-in-law until the rows prior to their impending divorce precipitated a big attack so that she was forced to leave and find accommodation of her own, and Mrs D finally left her husband when the worry of his compulsive gambling got to the stage where it was affecting her health.

Not all methods of pain control involve the same costs as restrictions in activity or the minimization of life stress since some were derived from observed connections between fluctuations in levels of pain and more mundane matters such as the weather.

> *Mrs V:* Now I got up this morning and I could hardly move and as soon as I looked out of me bedroom window I see it was wet and I thought 'Ah well, there's the answer.'

These causal theories are of intrinsic and extrinsic value for they offer a solution to the cognitive problem of finding meaning in experience and the practical problem constituted by the symptoms of the disease. On the basis of such theories all of the respondents tried not to get cold or wet and invested considerable financial resources in heating their homes and keeping warm.

Although the day-to-day fluctuations in levels of pain were largely a mystery, the need to be able to make sense of experience and thereby provide for the possibility of control meant that they were usually accounted for by reference to antecedent events of the kind documented above. These explanations were routinely invoked in spite of the fact that they did not always precede days in which the pain was particularly bad. Major and prolonged flare-ups were even more difficult to come to terms with, partly because there was no predictable end to such suffering and

partly because these episodes were even more difficult to tie to antecedent events. Because Mrs X was unable to find a reason for her flare-ups she could only conclude, 'I suppose it's in your blood and it just comes out.' In the face of this kind of uncertainty the person is left powerless to influence his or her future and can do nothing but hope. As Mrs X continued, 'It seems to be sort of lying dormant now so I'm just keeping my fingers crossed.'

An additional problem which adds to the distress of people attempting to cope with the symptoms of rheumatoid arthritis is that the pain itself is an ambiguous indicator of the course of the disease. Sudden increases or decreases in pain could be read as nothing more than the normal variation of pain levels or taken to be indicative of a longer-term improvement or decline. This was particularly the case where changes were sustained over a period of days. The uncertainty surrounding these changes allowed increases in pain to be explained away, as not really heralding the beginning of another flare-up, and decreases in pain to be interpreted as the beginning of a long hoped-for remission. Hopes thus raised were frequently dashed as the situation developed. In the two weeks prior to the second interview, Mrs N had been in a little more pain each day, and she was beginning to get worried. For the past two years she had been taking a combination of drugs that had kept her arthritis fairly quiescent, and having been through a very disabling acute phase she did not want 'to go back to the way I was'. During those two years she had had 'bad spells' every so often but they usually did not last so long. Throughout the interview, Mrs N tried to minimize the threat this new development posed by finding numerous explanations to normalize the experience: 'Maybe I'm getting a cold and it's making the joints ache'; 'Maybe I've got used to the tablets and they're no longer working'; 'I've been doing too much'; 'It's probably just a little spasm that will wear off'; 'In the last few weeks I've had a lot of different company; Perhaps I've overdone it, I must go back to the old routine.' She also tried to minimize the extent of the change itself; while the pain was now at a point where she could not face getting up in the morning, 'I went to the opticians today so it can't be *that* bad.' The ambiguous meaning of this development in her symptoms was not entirely resolved by these causal theories, and there was nothing for it but to wait and see what happened in order that the situation could be assessed in the light of accumulating evidence. While the uncertainty allowed her to maintain a degree of hope, 'It's probably just a phase I'm going through', it did begin to undermine her hopes for her long-term future: 'I thought I was getting better. You hear of a lot of cases where it just disappears, so I'm wondering what this is.'

Mrs T was also the victim of uncertainty. At her second interview she was in the midst of a severe and exceptionally painful attack that had not abated after nine months and whose course had proved difficult to read.

Consequently, she was also beginning to have doubts about her future.

> *Mrs T:* It does seem to be slightly improving but I've had four or five false starts in that respect over the last six months where for a week or maybe ten days I'm lulled into a false sense of security of thinking, 'Hello it's burnt itself out now for a time and things are going to start picking up.' And it's come back again. It's been an extremely difficult period, very frustrating and a little bit frightening because there's the slight fear that this time it's not going to go away, that it's just going to stay with me now and build and build.

Certain and uncertain trajectories

As Strauss (1975) has discussed, some diseases have fairly certain trajectories, either because they are non-progressive and little change may be expected over time, or because their phases and the relative rate at which those phases change can be anticipated. For individuals with diseases of this kind, planning and preparation can be made in advance so that the challenge of each new phase can be adequately met. This is not the case with rheumatoid arthritis. Not only do coping strategies and social arrangements have to be modified on a day-to-day basis, the uncertainty surrounding longer-term prospects means that planning for the future can be a hazardous enterprise. Any arrangements that are made may prove to be inadequate in the light of future developments. Such uncertain trajectories help to maximize the hardship experienced by the person with rheumatoid arthritis and his or her family.

In the face of uncertainty concerning long-term prospects, some of the respondents chose to cling to the possibility that the disease would burn out eventually so that a return to something akin to a normal existence was possible, while some had come to accept that they would deteriorate to such an extent that residential care would be necessary. An example of the former was Mr S. He had seen the pain progressively disappear from the joints in the top half of his body and was waiting for the pains in his legs to subside: 'It's just the last two joints now.' Consequently, he was looking forward to being able to return to work. An example of the latter was Mrs O. In spite of the fact that she said 'You never know how you'll be with arthritis', she accepted that her fate was one of long-term decline into dependency: 'I know as I get older it'll get worse, it's bound to. I've told my family that when I become a burden I want to go into a home.' Similarly, Mr H, bed-ridden and virtually helpless, was so pessimistic about his future that he no longer planned for himself but for his wife: 'It's just borrowed time before I'm boxed up.'

Mr S and Mrs O were both able to perceive a pattern in the past and present which allowed them to construct an image of the future and possible arrangements for coping with it. Neither, however, was in a position which required them to make decisions and radically reorganize their daily existence. Though certain of her eventual decline into total invalidity, Mrs O was able to say 'I feel, well, wait till that time comes along, as long as I can carry on like I am.' Their certainty provided for a knowable and controllable future and went unchallenged because it did not have to be transformed into action. By contrast, Mrs G faced an uncertain future while having reached a stage where she felt something had to be done to remedy what had become an intolerable situation. As well as having rheumatoid arthritis she was blind, diabetic, and also suffered another painful condition which had been diagnosed as polyneuritis. Just recently, and to her great distress, she had lost the sense of touch in her fingers and was no longer able to read braille. For the past year she had been virtually housebound because of pain and, despite having received all possible aids and appliances, her days were a nightmare of attempting to cope alone in her flat. When interviewed she said 'I can't drag myself around anywhere, this time I'm at the end of my tether.' She was upset because nothing her doctors did seemed to relieve the pain and also because they seemed reluctant to specify a prognosis. She had come to the conclusion that they were withholding information from her at a time when she needed to be told the truth in order to make rational decisions about possible future arrangements.

> *Mrs G:* I want to know what are my chances of getting better because if there isn't I've got to sit and think. I've got to do something else because I can't go on dragging myself around here indefinitely. If this isn't getting better then the person who's got to know about it is me 'cus I've got to make other arrangements. I have to look after myself, when I get back here I'm on my own, mate, so if I have to do something else . . . 'cus he said it'll take a long time, you know. Well, how long? Is it getting better? Is there a chance of it getting better? The next logical step for me is a residential home but it's no good me going into a home and then find in a year I'm better because once I give this flat up there's no way back. I don't want to find myself in a home at 55 where the people are 105 which is what would happen.

By the time the interviewing was completed, Mrs G was still trying to clarify her medical status and find some way of securing relief from pain and improved mobility. She was left with the dilemma of choosing between striving to maintain her independence or giving up the fight and going into a home. Because her condition was unpredictable, it was not clear which of these options would enhance the quality of her daily life.

Socio-psychological strategies of coping

The strategies that people with rheumatoid arthritis come to adopt as a result of their disease, its symptoms, and consequences can be categorized into a number of types. On the one hand there are strategies designed to cope with the practical problems created by disability (see Chapter 4), and on the other, strategies designed to manage the interactional problems chronically sick persons may encounter in their relations with others (see Chapter 6). It is also possible to identify a range of strategies by means of which they organize their response to the disease itself. Wiener has referred to these as socio-psychological strategies of tolerating (Wiener 1975). Wiener's analysis was largely concerned with the way in which people with rheumatoid arthritis tolerate uncertainty by 'juggling the hope of relief and/or remission against the dread of progression' (1975:99). Essentially, this balance of hope and dread allows the person to manage a problematic future. At the same time they must also manage a problematic present dominated by the certainty that they have a painful and disabling disorder for which there is no cure. This is achieved by another balance of opposites, *accepting it* and *living with it* at the same time as *fighting it* and *keeping going*. The demands they place on themselves and the demands placed on them by others are, then, somewhat contradictory; they must learn to be disabled people at the same time as learning how to limit their disability.

Like the people interviewed by Wiener, the people in this study had a dual orientation towards the future. They knew that the disease was progressive and could eventually lead to almost total invalidity, and such knowledge was reinforced when they came into contact with others who were more severely disabled. Seeing others who were worse off than themselves was something of a mixed blessing and gave rise to both gratitude and fear. On the one hand it made the present a little more tolerable:

> *Mrs I:* The people at this rehabilitation centre were quite deformed, it was heartbreaking. I thought 'We don't know how lucky he (Mr I) is,' although he is in pain and all that I felt like saying to him 'Don't complain, look at all these poor people here.'

On the other hand it rendered the future problematic by bringing with it the dread of progression and the dread of dependency:

> *Mrs N:* What if I go back to the way I was and end up in a wheelchair. I would hate that sort of thing. I'd rather be dead in other words, rather than be dependent upon others to wheel me about in a wheelchair and that sort of thing.

While life was often redesigned in order to control the symptoms of rheumatoid arthritis, it was also reorganized so as to minimize the chances of progression and dependency. In the case of Miss L, the same regimen functioned to achieve both of these goals. She rested in order to reduce pain and tried to keep active in order to keep the joints and muscles working: 'It doesn't cure you it keeps you mobile and if you're mobile you're not a burden.'

Life regimens such as that adopted by Miss L did not guarantee that the disease would not progress until it finally resulted in helplessness. Even where it appeared to have stabilized, there was no certainty that the disease *had* been arrested by these or other efforts. As Miss L finally commented after discussing her attempts to avoid invalidity, 'You can't tell with this, you never know, it's never gone away forever.' Under these circumstances all that remained was hope, either the hope for remission or, at least, relief (Wiener 1975). For Mrs A this was the simple hope that the disease would disappear on its own: 'I'm always hopeful that one day I'll wake up and it'll all have gone away', while for Mrs G it was the hope that with courage and energy she could return to some semblance of health:

> *Mrs G:* The book says it's progressive, but I don't believe that, at least I don't want to. I'm still hoping to fight my way back.

Mr F hoped that medical intervention would eventually restore him to something approaching normal functioning, 'You hear about people in the same predicament as me having operations and getting well', and he knew of several people who had had joints replaced and were fit enough to go back to work. His long-term strategy was to move out of London so that he could attend a hospital where he believed these operations were performed as a matter of routine, and he became very critical of the doctors at the hospital he currently attended who did not seem to be prepared to help in this way. By contrast, Mrs T did not entertain the hope of recovery, merely the hope that something might be done to relieve her of pain. She continued to hope that someone would come up with a drug effective against arthritis, and hope had been rekindled when she was told that her application to the local authority to be rehoused would be dealt with as a priority. This meant that she would finally have access to a bath.

> *Mrs T:* It has been a tremendous encouragement to know that we're not at the bottom of the list and something *will* be done. The only thing is I hope they get a move on because the bathing business, the immersion in warm water, does give you a temporary benefit. I've sat for hours with my hands in warm water, it's very comforting. I feel that there *is* something in the future that's going to help.

In this way hope not only counters the dread of progression and dependency but also helps to make the present a little more tolerable.

While the future is problematic to the person with a chronic illness, the present is even more so since it involves coming to terms with a reduction in activity as well as the often distressing symptoms of the particualr disorder. All of the respondents in this study had at some time been told that they could not be cured and that their only option was to learn to live with arthritis, adjusting their life'so as to conform to the demands of the disease. Learning to live with rheumatoid arthritis not only required that ways be developed of performing activities of daily living in spite of pain and stiffness, it also required that limited activity and constant discomfort were accepted as their lot in life. For some, coming to terms with chronic illness provided an escape from the emotional torment that followed the onset of invalidity.

> *Mrs A:* When it first happened I got quite neurotic about it . . . very neurotic and very difficult. You know, why this has happened to me? and, I can't go on living like this. But you get over it. I think if you can accept it it's a great thing and if you can accept your limitations it's a great thing too.

In many ways this strategy of accepting is similar to the process of re-normalization described by Reif (1973). It consists of changing personal values and lowering expectations to match the reduction in physical capacity attendant upon rheumatoid arthritis. It involves lowering standards of performance to bring them in line with limited mobility and reserves of energy which are rapidly exhausted, and it means being content to operate within new and narrowed boundaries of activity. For the arthritic, a 'good day' is not a day without pain but a day with normal pain. *Accepting it* means abandoning an unattainable normality and replacing it with a reconstructed normality which allows for gratification, satisfaction, and a sense of achievement. Consequently, the mundane activities of everyday life, taken for granted by the non-impaired, take on extraordinary significance. For example, Mrs R, who was becoming increasingly housebound, was able to derive a sense of achievement and enormous satisfaction out of the simple activity of accompanying her daughter to the local shop.

> *Mrs R:* We love it, you know, even if we only go round to Tesco's. To us, you know, we get a terrific lot of pleasure which I think is good if you can find pleasure that way.

Similarly, Mrs O found value in doing household chores, ' 'cus I talk to myself, when I've done a job I say "There you are, that's good, you've done that." '

There was some evidence to suggest that an invalid status was more readily accepted by those who had been disabled for a number of years and by those whose condition had remained stable. Mr S had been disabled since his early twenties and claimed to be quite happy with things in general: 'I know I'm limited so I don't overdo it and that's all I can do.' By contrast, Mrs A had been limited for a little over five years and was constantly striving to maintain as broad a range of activities as possible: 'I can always think of things I ought to be trying to do.' The problem faced by people with a progressive disease is that they may constantly, or at least periodically, be called upon to adjust to reductions in physical capacity, what Wiener referred to as 'spiral re-normalisation into lower and lower expectations' (1975:101), as each flare-up left them with additional damage to the joints and higher residual levels of pain. This may take them below a level they judge to be acceptable and may call into question their ability to adjust.

> *Mrs J:* I've got it, I'm not going to get rid of it, so I've got to get on with it and that is the way I accept arthritis, except that I don't accept it because I won't. You see, arthritis is a painful thing so you grow to accept that. The pain doesn't worry me too much now, I just say a few expletives and carry on with what I'm doing. It's the incapacity that gets on my nerves, the pain doesn't. I can cope with the pain, it's the not being able to do things that causes me problems.

This ambiguity between accepting and not accepting the presence of a limiting disorder derives in part from the contradictory situation in which people with rheumatoid arthritis find themselves. While they recognize the necessity of accepting their lot in life and ceasing to berate fate for their misfortune, they also recognize the necessity of not succumbing to the disease. Consequently, they must 'carry on', 'keep going', and 'get on with it' despite the pain and discomfort this involves. Many told stories of people they knew who had retired to bed and become totally dependent upon others for all their needs, so they fought to find the courage and the energy to maintain some level of activity. This strategy of keeping going is quite distinct from the strategy described by Wiener as keeping-up; it is not an attempt to maintain normal levels of activity but an attempt to perform any activity in order to prevent stagnation and further loss of faculty. Even the most severely disabled in this group of people tried to keep going in some respects, no matter how minimal the activity in which they engaged, in order to prevent their lives from being totally dominated by pain.

> *Mrs R:* As long as I can keep going. Even if I just drive Carol as far as round the corner to the shop I've achieved something.

Mrs J came closest to keeping-up, but even here she was as much concerned with keeping going in order to prevent what was perceived as the all-too-easy slide into the static existence of the invalid. Despite having five grown-up children living at home, she insisted on continuing to do the housework.

> *Mrs J:* Every time I stop doing something it's one more thing I can't do. Take my washing, if it kills me I'll do it because if I stop doing it that's one more thing I can't do. I scrubbed me kitchen on me hands and knees Thursday. It crippled me but that's beside the point, I shall still do it because once again if I don't do it it's something else I can't do. If I didn't, I feel that eventually I shall finish up getting out of bed, walking downstairs, sitting here all day and then at night walking back up again and I'm not prepared to do that!

Some effort was often invested in maintaining key activities without which the quality of life would decline dramatically. Mrs R was confined to a wheelchair so the ability to drive made an enormous difference to her mobility around the community.

> *Mrs R:* I couldn't get from my chair into my car one day and that panicked me, so I made myself keep trying and trying and well, now I try not to let a day miss, even if it just means sliding from the chair into the car to make myself do it and it has been a bit easier, you know, it's just sort of keeping going. This is the main thing, to keep going.

Keeping going and doing something, in fact anything, is of value for a number of reasons. Firstly, it is a source of exercise and means that muscles and joints are being used and prevented from deteriorating to a stage where they cannot be used. In fact, many wished they could go swimming in order to keep mobile but few did since the facilities available were inaccessible, too expensive or so far away that the pain of getting there and back outweighed any benefit to be gained. Secondly, keeping going was of psychological and symbolic value in that it was indicative of their ability to continue to fight the disease and its effects. It is for this reason that some refused to use a walking stick or take sleeping tablets at night since these were indicative of 'giving in'. Consequently, though many often wanted to avoid the pain and effort of getting through the day by staying in bed, few did. Unless forced upon them by a particularly severe flare-up, such behaviour was taken to be a moral lapse. When I asked Mrs R if she ever spent the whole day in bed she said 'I wouldn't like to tell you, I get so ashamed. Sometimes I've stayed in bed for a whole week through no reason, just 'cus I couldn't be bothered to get up, which is very bad.' Similarly, Mrs T tried to avoid spending any part of the day in bed.

> *Mrs T:* I think it's psychologically bad because if you continually do something it becomes a habit and then you start adopting the attitude that you can't do anything else. You get to the point where you say 'I

must go to bed in the afternoon' and if someone says 'Why must you?' it's 'Well, I always do.' That's no good at all.

In this way invalidity was perceived by some very much as a state of mind which could easily take over and precipitate a rapid decline into helplessness. In fighting rheumatoid arthritis they were often fighting both the disease and themselves, and it was only their own psychological resources that allowed them to retain some independence in the face of chronic pain and loss of energy. As Mrs X said, 'It's up to me to sort of keep going, isn't it?'

Stragegies of *accepting it* and *keeping going* did, of course, break down. This often happened during an acute phase when unremitting pain made any activity virtually impossible because the sheer effort of coping with the pain drained already depleted resources of energy. Then, giving up altogether and staying in bed was virtually all that could be done. By the time of the second interview, Mrs T had been in severe pain for nigh on nine months and was now spending the majority of the day in bed in spite of her misgivings about such a course of action.

> *Mrs T:* I don't necessarily think this is a good thing either psychologically or physically to do this but it's where I get the most comfort so it's a bit difficult to become a martyr and say 'No I'm not going back to bed I'm going to stay up' when, you know, just to go in and lie down is more comfortable.

Episodes like this were, however, regarded as temporary lapses and frequently gave rise to requests to doctors for 'something to ease the pain and get me going again'. Equally temporary were the lapses that arose when the day-to-day grind became too much. At one interview Miss B was able to say 'People say to me "You've got all this, you've had all these operations and you're laughing and joking." I said "Well, there's no good moping, is there? There's no good in giving way" ', while at the next she said 'The other night I felt like crying my eyes out, my friend had come up and she said "What's the matter with you?" "Oh," I said "I'm depressed." "Well," she says "you've got to live with it." "Oh," I said "don't keep telling me that." '

Other breakdowns in these coping strategies were more permanent and represented another step in the downward drift towards dependence and helplessness. The process of getting ready to go out gradually became too much trouble so social activities were curtailed, activities previously undertaken alone were now undertaken only in the presence of others, and tasks such as household chores given over entirely to relatives, friends, or formal helpers. While regrettable, this inability to keep going at the same pace was often the consequence of ageing or the sheer duration of the disease; sometimes the individual became burnt out before the arthritis. Mrs R and Mrs G had been arthritic since their early twenties and had worked and brought up families in spite of unhappy and unsupportive marriages and long spells in hospitals or convalescent homes. Mrs R's life had been 'a terrific fight' but now, 'I've got to the stage where I can't fight it like I used to. When I was younger I'd do anything to get out and get going but I've got to the stage where I have given in a bit.' With Mrs G, giving up coincided with a gradual loss of hope. At the first interview she still regarded her complex medical problems as a challenge and believed that by her own efforts she would fight her way back to mobility and independence as she had many times in the past: 'I like to think I can still win and pull it out of the fire just once more simply because I don't fancy sitting here for the next 20 years.' One year later, after the failure of her many attempts to secure co-operation from her doctors and with no improvement in her condition, she was having to consider residential care: 'I've just come to the end of the road; even I can't fight it anymore.' As she added at the end of the interview, 'I find I'm coming to the end of even my inner resources. You can only take so much pain and it's been going on for some years. I'm not talking about weeks and months, I'm talking about *years*.' Without incentives such as hope, work or family responsibilities, the struggle to keep going became meaningless and more difficult to sustain.

Such changes do of course, have implications for identity, particularly when it seems that the ability to win out over the disease is lost. In this case, keeping cheerful, or finding some humour in the face of a desperate situation, provide a last resort by which people with a disabling illness can retain integrity and demonstrate to others that, no matter how incapacitated, they are not entirely beaten by the disease. For Mr H, bed-bound and breathless, a sense of humour was virtually all that remained.

> *Mr H:* I think one has to have a sense of humour about these things or all you can do is chuck it in all together. I'm a cynic, I've always said the whole of life is just a preparation for death. But you can have a sense of humour about it. I had a laugh the other day. I was down in the nursing unit and there's a man down there sitting in the lounge with me and he's got one of these communicators, I don't know if you've seen them, strapped to his wrist, a sort of little typewriter thing. So he's tapping out the message you see to me and trying to give me the tape and he's sitting there and can't move from his chair and his hand is shaking like this and I'm sitting here and can't move from my chair and trying to reach over for the tape and my hand's shaking. I'm trying to get it like this and he's trying to give it to me. Talk about ridiculous! We can't get the tape over between us, you see. The only thing is, you can have a sense of humour.

Vulnerability and insecurity

As well as organizing their lives in a manner which controls symptoms and minimizes the impact of their disorder, rheumatoid arthritics must also come to terms with their own vulnerability, whether actual or perceived. Given weak joints, stiff and unresponsive limbs, and a general instability while standing or walking, the everyday world becomes fraught with danger. Because arthritic joints have a habit of suddenly giving way or provide inadequate support, the physical environment constitutes a hazard, while ordinary activities are a source of danger. Travelling on a bus, walking across a room, or cooking a meal may be avoided altogether or are carefully planned so as to reduce the risk of injury. In the face of this fear of and susceptibility to injury, ordinary everyday objects and events take on an alarming character and may give rise to feelings of insecurity equally as disabling as the impairment itself. This perceived vulnerability sometimes disabled the spouse and sometimes the entire family. This happened where the individual was defined by others as incapable of being left alone.

Mr H was the most severely disabled person interviewed for the study and was virtually bedridden, having an as yet undiagnosed respiratory condition which often left him breathless as well as active arthritis which had produced a high degree of deformity in his limbs. He could do little for himself and was totally dependent upon his wife who rarely left him alone. They had few social contacts and Mrs H went out only to get the shopping. Even that proved to be a major problem.

> *Mrs H:* I'd think 'Is he all right on is own? Is there anything he'll want?' And I was at the stage I was running to the shops and running back and if there was a queue I would leave it because I knew he was on his own.

This had imposed such a strain on Mrs H that, with the help of their doctor, they were allocated a flat in a block specially constructed for the severely disabled. Attached was a nursing unit where Mr H could be left if his wife needed to be out for any length of time, and there was a bell in the flat which could be used to summon the nurses if help was required in an emergency. Because getting Mr H out of bed, dressed and down to the nursing unit was an enterprise in itself, Mrs H would leave him alone with the bell if all she wanted to do was shop. This limited her to the relatively expensive local shops since taking advantage of the supermarkets in the High Street would mean she was away from the flat for more than an hour.

Mr I was nowhere near as disabled as Mr H; while his ability to walk was limited he was able to get around indoors without help, yet the fear that he might fall imposed rigorous constraints on the other members of his family.

Mrs I: I keep my children off school sometimes, I say 'You've got to stay with daddy. I've got to go here or there today.' It's just not fair to the children 'cus you've got to keep somebody here all the time. There is that possibility he could fall and he'd never be able to get up.

Again, simple everyday activities like shopping were a major problem since being out of the house meant having the constant worry that Mr I might suffer an accident or otherwise be in need of help. As a result of this fear, Mrs I gradually became as housebound as Mr I. The problem was eased somewhat when Mr I was given aids to help with bathing; once in the bath he was felt to be relatively secure, and Mrs I would then leave him to go out to the shops.

Mrs I: While he's in the bath I can run across the road 'cus I know full well he's not going to fall 'cus he's got a slip mat in there and he's got the thing that he sits on. I know now he's not going to fall and I can go across to the shop a little bit clear headed, I haven't got to worry where before I just couldn't leave. If the children were at school I'd have to make sure he was sitting down and say don't get up I'll just pop over the road and get the dinner, you know. I'd do it in record time, you daren't be out any longer. I mean, you had to run to the shops, you daren't stop and talk to a friend because I've got to get in. I mean, you just couldn't stand and talk to nobody. You know, come in shut your door and carry on life from there.

Nearly all of the respondents talked about their fear of falling at some stage during the interviewing since it carried the risk of injury or the possibility that they would be left lying on the floor or in the road unable to get up. Not all had fallen, and of those who had, few had actually been hurt. Nevertheless, all organized themselves in such a way so as to minimize the chances that they would fall or do themselves a damage if they did. Mr P had arranged the furniture in his flat so that if he did feel he was going to fall, there was always something nearby he could catch onto and steady himself. Cupboards and book shelves were placed at strategic points along the major routes around his flat to support him as he moved from room to room. Other than that the spaces were kept clear in order to avoid the possibility of tripping on objects scattered around the room and to provide a relatively safe landing should his legs give way. In moving about parts of his flat where there was nothing on which to hold, he always used his stick which helped prevent his falling and helped him to get up if he did. In the lounge was a small stool and in the bathroom, the scene of many falls, he kept pieces of wood and used these to gradually work his way back to his feet. Mrs K frequently got up during the night and because Mr K felt there was a greater chance of her falling while half asleep, the lounge was always cleared of furniture which had hard edges and sharp corners, leaving only the soft furnishings which could do her no harm.

Mr K appeared to believe that his wife was so vulnerable and in such danger that his protective strategies all but excluded her from participation in household affairs.

> *Mr K:* You see, I won't let her touch anything that's hot, saucepans or kettles, because it only needs a slight twist and she could do herself a bad injury. Well, I wouldn't want that so, you see, I must take steps to prevent it happening. It's the same with an iron, you see. She tries doing little bits from time to time but when it comes to big things she's inclined to get a bit flustered, she'd knock the iron over and panic and that sort of thing and when she comes to turn round she nearly falls over.

Bathing was another ordinary activity perceived as a possible source of danger and always accompanied by the fear of slipping on wet floors or in the bath itself. Nearly all had acquired or improvised aids to prevent their slipping, and few would take a bath if they were alone. Mrs A had fallen several times in the bath and got to the stage where 'I was afraid to get in.' Having acquired aids, she said, 'I'm not in the least bothered but I never have a bath unless someone's around and the door is always left slightly open.' Of those who lived alone, some did not bath at all and some only bathed when they went to visit relatives.

Although the propensity to fall makes the domestic environment a source of danger, the threat can be reduced by modifications in the layout and character of the home. Not so the community at large. Here the disabled person must learn to live with hazards that are largely outside his or her control. Again, the fear of falling was predominant, partly because of the additional risks posed by uneven pavements and the like and partly because objects were not always readily at hand to provide a source of support. In addition, falls in public carried the risk of symbolic as well as physical injury. Mr C had fallen many times in the street:

> *Mr C:* I can get up if I can grab something. If nothing is convenient that's when it's worse, you're in trouble then if you can't get near anything to help you to get up and even if I did I sometimes haven't the strength to lift me up anyway.
> *Int:* What do you do then?
> *Mr C:* Well, I get a hand, there are plenty of people will give you a hand but others won't, they just walk by, probably they think you're drunk if they see you lying there and you can't get up.

One experience had made Mr C very wary of zebra crossings: 'I did fall there once and I tell you it's scary lying there in the road seeing the cars coming at you.'

The risks posed by pavements that were not well maintained and the desire to avoid the embarrassment of having to be picked up on the street were often sufficient to keep people at home. Miss B would walk as far as the main door of the block of flats in which she lived but no further:'They tell me it's uneven out there', and having fallen once just outside his house Mr F did not want the indignity of falling in front of others so only went out in order to keep hospital appointments. For those who did continue to go out getting around the immediate community required vigilance and planning. Prominent paving stones and things like wet leaves have to be spotted in advance and carefully negotiated since slipping, stumbling, or catching the feet on uneven surfaces created pain even if it did not result in a fall. Snow and ice were particularly dangerous and if they did not lead to confinement required additional care. If it had snowed Mrs J only went out in the late afternoon and walked in the middle of the road where the cars had by that time cleared a path. Using public transport also carried a risk. Mr C had been slow to get off an underground train and had been trapped in the automatic doors. He never used it again. Mrs A had fallen once or twice after having to stand on full buses and now tolerated the frustration of waiting for a bus to arrive which had vacant seats relatively close to the door. In this way, some of the respondents attempted to remain mobile and safe in a world that was not structured in a manner favourable to their physical needs.

The selective allocation of resources

One problem common to many, if not all, chronically sick individuals is that of constructing an acceptable kind of life using radically reduced resources. Time, money, physical strength, energy, and social contacts may all shrink as a result of the illness and its disabling effects. Consequently, the person is constantly called upon to make choices concerning how these instrumentalities are to be used and must try to allocate them in a manner such that the maximum is gained from what is still available. In some cases choices may be made on the basis of personal values; at other times there may be a little real choice at all. People living alone may decide not to expend valuable energy on cleaning the house, but if they cannot get out to do the shopping they may have to use their limited income to pay someone to do it. Otherwise they do not eat. In this way, different resources may be given over to different tasks so that the sum total adds up to 'managing to get by'.

Fagerhaugh (1973) has described this process with respect to emphysema sufferers whose main difficulty is in getting enough oxygen to furnish the energy to perform everyday activities. A person with normal lungs can do a number of activities at the same time; the emphysema patient cannot. They must select how they will use their limited oxygen supply and postpone other activities until energy has been replenished. A similar problem faces the person with rheumatoid arthritis, particularly during acute phases when supplies of energy are largely exhausted by the effort of coping with pain. Then they must preserve what remains in order that it be used for essential or valued activities. A good example of this was Mrs T who, during the flare-up described previously, chose to spend most of the day in bed, partly because it was more comfortable there and partly because it required little energy.

> *Mrs T:* If it's not a day when my home help comes I'll get up, make some tea and I'll go back and stay in bed for the rest of the day so that what little energy I have got I'll be able to use when my husband comes home to make two or three pleasant hours for both of us. And when I say both of us I look forward to that period tremendously which obviously is the peak of my day when he comes home, so naturally when he comes home I want to feel as good as I can.

Even participating in the interview consumed energy which then had to be restored before further activity could take place.

> *Mrs T:* You see, the upshot of our conversation this afternoon, I hope it isn't coming over to you as such, but to talk to you as I have is a tremendous effort and it's because I think I'm interested in what you're doing is the only thing keeping me going and when you've gone I'll sort of go 'Uh!' And I'll have to go to bed.

The selective allocation of physical resources is not confined to the acute phases of the disease; it is also a demand placed on the person even when his or her arthritis is relatively quiescent. Here choices have to be made because of the body's limited tolerance to activity and the need to preserve another valuable resource, the integrity of the joints. For example, those who have rheumatoid arthritis rapidly learn that only so much activity per day is possible before pain increases to unacceptable levels. The day's quota must then be given over to a small number of valued or necessary tasks and the remainder given up altogether or left for another day. Mrs N allowed herself one walk a day after which she would need to rest for two hours for the pain the walk produced to subside. She would normally use the walk to do her shopping but on the day of the first interview, she had an appointment with an optician and had to reserve the walk for that. The desire to prevent further damage to the joints also led some individuals to maintain some activities at the expense of others. Miss L used to do a lot of dressmaking and knitting: 'I don't do anything like that now, I'd rather keep my hands for when I work.' Some managed their limited physical resources in a manner similar to that described by Wiener (1975) as pacing, learning what one is able to do, how often, and in what manner. Until her daughter left school and took responsibility for household affairs, Mrs R used to get through her housework by doing a little, resting, doing a little more, and resting again until the jobs were finally done.

Another resource the chronically sick person may have to allocate very carefully is that of time. For those who have rheumatoid arthritis time appears to shrink, partly because so much is taken up by resting and partly because each task takes so long to complete that very little may be achieved in what is left. As Mrs A said, 'You always get there in the end but it just takes a very long time.' For most of the time she could only walk very slowly, and as she lived on the top floor of a block of flats without a lift, it took ten minutes or more for her to climb down fifty-two steps. Going out meant leaving home especially early if she was to make sure she arrived at the appointed time. This necessity of allocating disproportionate amounts of time to ordinary activities was a continual source of frustration.

Mrs A: You always feel you're a little bit behind. At the end of the day there's always a load you meant to do and could never quite manage.

For those who worked a very early start was necessary to make sure they got to the office on time. Prior to her retirement Mrs A was up at five so that she could be certain of being mobile enough to get a bus and arrive at work by 9.30. Miss L was always very slow in getting washed and dressed and was always up by 6.30: 'I can't do these things in a rush, I must have time.' Her mornings were always tightly scheduled and there was little room for flexibility.

Miss L: I'm a creature of routine now. I *must* get up at 6.30. If I stay in bed ten minutes longer I can't make it up by hurrying.

When time is so necessary to complete everyday tasks, any interruption can upset the schedule and means the task has to be abandoned. If Mrs R wished to go out, then she and her daughter had to get up early and get her ready: 'Then the phone goes and perhaps I'm on a long time, well by that time the clock has gone round and I think "Well, what's the good now by the time she's got me washed, dressed and out it isn't going to be worth it." '

Becoming disabled

Learning how to pace activities and cope with greatly diminished resources is part of a broader process which may be referred to as *becoming disabled*. People with a chronic illness not only have to learn how to manage symptoms, medical crises, and therapeutic regimens (Strauss 1975), they also have to learn to live with physical limitations. This

involves discovering new ways of performing everyday tasks and discovering which tasks cannot be done or should not be attempted. Miss L
encapsulated this process very nicely when she said 'Really, it's finding
what you can do and finding your limitations and not trying to be too
ambitious.'

This process of becoming disabled is facilitated in two ways; firstly, by
the advice given by doctors or co-sufferers and secondly, by personal
experience. It is largely by trial and error that the boundaries of activity
are defined and periodically reaffirmed and meaning given to advice
previously provided. For example, shortly after diagnosis Mr I was told
that there was no cure for his condition and the only way to prevent
further deterioration was complete rest: 'He said "It's no good you trying
to walk a mile every day or anything like that." He said "You've got to rest
your joints and that is it." ' What this meant in practice emerged over the
next few months as various activities were attempted and found to be
beyond him. He tried walking from his home to his doctor's surgery, just
over a mile away, 'I left at nine and got back at ten to one, you know, just
going down to the doctor's and back again. I had to stop, then start, then
stop.' When asked if he would be able to use public transport if
accompanied by his wife he said 'we wouldn't try', and told how he went
with his wife by bus to the local shopping centre but had been unable to
climb onto the bus to get back. Finally, he attempted to walk round to his
local pub instead of waiting for friends to arrive with a car: 'We was only
half way round and I couldn't go any further. We just stood there hoping
they was on their way round which they were and they picked us up out
here and that's just from here to the gate round there.' These and other
similar experiences helped Mr I to define the limits of his world; he
remained confined to the house and only went out if transport could be
arranged. At the time of the interviewing, he could only conceive of a
return to a more extensive social existence if a cure could be found for his
disease. Similar experiences acted as critical incidents, transforming
identities, definitions of self and, ultimately, life chances. After two
operations and ten months in hospital, Mrs X attempted to regain some of
her previous mobility. Twice she went out with her daughters and
despite having gone only a short distance, she was in such pain that they
had to take a taxi home. Consequently, 'I got it into my head, "Oh well,
you're not going to get out and walk about that's obvious" ' and was more
or less housebound for the next seven years, five of which she spent in a
wheelchair. It was only through the determination of her family that she
had recently begun to walk again.

In view of the fluctuating character of rheumatoid arthritis, these
boundaries to activity have constantly to be learned and relearned. Each
acute phase is followed by a period in which the tolerance to activity is
tested, while extended periods of remission give rise to a sense of security

which stimulates further testing. Where such experimentation proves to be disastrous, it may merely reaffirm the extent of the disability; on the other hand, it may modify the boundary by revealing the conditions under which the activity needs to be performed. One afternoon Mrs N decided to clean her oven but having finished the job she was unable to get back onto her feet and was forced to sit on the floor until someone came home to help her up. The experience was not without value for it contributed to her understanding of her limitations: 'I won't do that again, get down *with no one in the house.*'

Note

1. Rheumatism and arthritis are terms commonly applied to any pain located in bones, muscles, or joints, whatever its origin. Rheumatoid arthritis, however, is a distinct clinical entity and a disease of the entire body system. It differs in this respect from osteoarthritis which is generally localized to weight bearing joints and is a degenerative disorder associated with ageing. The main feature of rheumatoid arthritis is inflammation of the synovial membrane which lines the joint cavity. As a result of inflammation this membrane thickens and grows, the joints swell and become acutely painful with high internal pressure. Enlargement of the joints causes the ligaments which hold the bones in place to stretch and weaken and the joint to deform and dislocate. The inflamed synovial membrane overgrows the cartilage in the joint and as this is progressively destroyed the exposed bone begins to erode. Gradually, the proliferating membrane fills the entire joint cavity so that movement is severely limited. Over time fibrous tissue appears binding all into a permanently stiffened and deformed joint. Tendon sheaths may also become inflamed and inflammatory nodules appear on pressure points in the hands and elbows. Other complications include anaemia, trapping of nerves in the knees and elbows, pleurisy, and a form of conjunctivitis. The main effect of these disease processes is a drastic reduction in mobility and ambulation. Unlike conditions such as paraplegia and multiple sclerosis where such reduction stems from destruction or degeneration of the nerve pathways controlling movement, the problem for the rheumatoid arthritis patient arises from damage to the joints themselves.

3 Medical care and therapeutic intervention

The lives of chronically sick and disabled people are intimately bound up with, if not dominated by, two major institutions of modern society, those of medicine and welfare. Accordingly, they become subject to the decisions of others who allocate them to clinical and administrative categories, define their needs and the most appropriate way of meeting them. The individual's view of his or her problems often does not match that of those who control the resources he or she seeks; nevertheless, in consulting professional providers, the individual loses responsibility for decisions concerning the illness and its effects and may have no choice but to accept the definitions imposed on him or her by others (Bloor and Horobin 1975).

The role of medical care in chronic illness is, of course, central. Doctors are usually the first experts that are consulted in the course of the illness career. They provide the clinical labels by which persons become officially chronically sick and signal the beginning of the process by which the disabled become segregated from society (Freidson 1965). They provide the cognitive resources which help to reduce pain and functional limitation, they are called upon to verify the disabled person's claims for benefits and services, and they have a significant impact on the illness career by influencing conceptions of self and defining appropriate conduct for the person concerned. Consequently, medical decision making is of some importance in the social processes which lead to the development of disability and handicap. For example, individuals may want to continue to work but become unemployed and dependent upon welfare payments at the insistence of their doctors whose prime interest is in enhancing the patient's clinical condition by therapeutic intervention and modification of life style. Some have argued that the influence of medicine has extended beyond clinical concerns to the point where it now dominates the administration of services and benefits for chronically sick and disabled people, an involvement which does not always operate in the best interests of the recipients (Blaxter 1976; Walker 1981).

To point out that the institutions of medicine and welfare operate with and impose definitions of need which may differ from those of their clients is not to claim that they are of no help. In this study many of the

respondents spoke highly of individual doctors, social workers, rehabilitation officers, and the like or praised their hospital or State or local social
service provision for the disabled. Even Mrs R, the most severe critic of
welfare agencies, said: 'These days the benefits are so good.' However,
while many problems are partially or wholly solved by these institutions,
many others are created which remain unsolved or consume time,
energy, or other scarce resources. As far as medical care is concerned,
these difficulties ranged from problems which emerge during contacts
with medical personnel to problems which are created by therapeutic
interventions which may be distressing or have undesirable side effects.
This chapter ignores the success stories in order to focus on these
problems.

The acquisition of a diagnosis

The careers of the twenty-four people interviewed for this study varied
widely. Some became rapidly disabled soon after onset, left work and
became housebound, while others experienced little disruption of their
lives for many years until an acute flare-up left them appreciably disabled.
Some deteriorated slowly and steadily over the years so that all they could
say was 'it's just got worse', while others experienced periods of stability
and sudden declines. The same degree of variation was also evident in the
very early stages of the illness career, that is between first symptoms and
diagnosis. In some, but not all, cases there was a gap of months or years
before what eventually came to be recognized as the initial manifestations
of the disease were labelled as rheumatoid arthritis, the gap having been
created by patient delay and mis-diagnosis of the early signs and
symptoms.

The timing of the first contact with a doctor and the timing of the
referral by the doctor to a specialist out-patient clinic depended upon the
nature and severity of the first symptoms and the speed with which they
had first developed. Symptoms which developed slowly or which could
be explained away by reference to some antecedent event, like a minor
accident or previous illness, were treated at home and did not give rise to
much concern. This was also the case where the pain was confined to one
joint, was intermittent and not too severe. When the symptoms developed to the stage where they did give rise to a consultation, diagnoses
were often given which indicated that nothing much was wrong, and this
sometimes created further delay because these diagnoses could be used
to explain subsequent bouts of pain. The case of Mr F provides a good
illustration of this process. He had been having pain in his wrists and
intermittent difficulty in gripping tools for two years before he sought
medical advice: 'I didn't think much about it at the time, you know, aches
and pains; I used to work a lot outside and we worked long hours and I

thought it was nothing serious. Nothing actually came on sudden with it.' He went to his doctor when pain began to appear in other parts of his body and was told that he had arthritis, 'he didn't say what type or anything like that', and was given tablets which eased the pain. Despite frequent pain it was another four years before he went back to his doctor: 'I went a very long time without bothering about it because I thought it was just one of those things, you know, ordinary arthritis and I didn't think it would get any worse. I had to go back to him in the end because it got so bad in the legs.'

As many studies have revealed, this prediagnostic phase can be a period of great distress (Burton 1975; Cunningham 1977; Locker 1981). This is particularly the case where the symptoms are vague or uncorroborated by external manifestations or where visits to doctors do not produce diagnoses to legitimate the personal experience of discomfort. In these cases the persons may find themselves labelled in a variety of derogatory ways or may come to doubt the reality of their experience. Where this happens the diagnosis, when finally given, is greeted with relief. Although Miss L recalled a number of episodes of pain and disability during adolescence, it was during her thirties that her problems began.

> *Miss L:* I was 37 when it came on with a bang. It wasn't so much pain but I felt very very tired and I went along to the hospital on my own bat and they did tests and said there was nothing wrong and I said 'I just don't understand why I feel so tired' and they said 'Just be glad there's nothing wrong with you.' So I thought 'Well, I must be imagining it, I must have a low threshold of pain because they couldn't find anything' and I started to get thinner and thinner and I went round to my doctor and he gave me Butazolidin and I had that for a long time and then I couldn't get round to that doctor my feet, everything was so very bad I could hardly walk . . . it took me two hours to get up in the morning and then they said at work 'we can't keep you here, you can't type and you're coming in so late.' But I couldn't give any reason, it had come on so slowly I didn't realize how incapacitated I was. Well, then I thought there really must be something wrong with me because, this may sound funny, but some people might have a low threshold of pain but it seemed so painful, so excruciatingly painful, it was everywhere, I couldn't do my hair, my fingers started swelling like bananas. I couldn't get round to my doctor I went to one nearer and he said 'You must go into hospital. You've got rheumatoid arthritis.' Funnily enough, I was glad someone told me because I thought 'I can't keep losing so much weight and looking so dreadful.' Once I knew I thought I could contend with it, I knew what I was battling with.

Even after diagnosis some felt that the reality of their symptoms continued to be questioned. Mrs G had a long, complex, and somewhat confusing medical history, the main feature of which seemed to be her continual difficulty to get her doctors to accept the reality of her complaints and to follow them up sufficiently to arrive at a diagnosis. Her initial complaints of severe pain in the back and legs had been diagnosed as 'psychological spine', and she had been sent away with analgesic and a spinal support: ' "Here's some pain killers, darling, it doesn't really exist, you're imagining it." ' At one stage she had been referred to a psychiatrist for investigation and felt stigmatized by her personal history as a Jewess who had fled Germany in the 1930s and had subsequently lost her entire family. She had been complaining of severe pain in her knees and legs, 'it feels as if the nerves are trapped', and found it too painful to stand or even walk. She felt her doctor's response had been one of ' "You should be all right, you're imagining things, why don't you get on with it, why don't you walk a bit more." I thought "If only you knew how sore I was you wouldn't make statements like that." ' She had only been given a diagnosis of polyneuritis when she was taken by mistake to the Casualty Department and saw a doctor there and not her consultant. She had recently lost the sense of touch in the fingers of her right hand and remembered complaining of strange sensations some years previously which were not followed up: 'People simply looked, couldn't see anything, didn't believe me, and left it.' Consequently, Mrs G was somewhat critical of the care she had received, and she must have been a difficult patient to manage both clinically and interactionally.

> *Mrs G:* Now they simply say 'We've got to a situation where this lady has four chronic conditions', which produces a little bit of a question mark in my head 'cus I think 'If I've been in your care all this time how on earth can any of them have got chronic, why didn't they get picked up?' Why is it when I say anything it falls on cloth ears?

However, in spite of her current distress and many complaints, she was able to appreciate the difficulties her case presented.

> *Mrs G:* As a nurse I find it a bit difficult to say things like that 'cus I know I could be very bitter and very annoyed with them. I also know that no doctor makes a wrong diagnosis deliberately, it simply wasn't picked up like so many things weren't picked up over the years. To diagnose a thing like this is probably a heck of a job anyway and there were so many other things wrong which took priority, they didn't know where to start.

The difficulties in diagnosing chronic conditions and the delay to which this may give rise can have an adverse effect on subsequent doctor-patient relationships. Even when patients are highly satisfied with the care they receive following diagnosis, the initial difficulties may leave some residual resentment. Mrs J first went to her doctor complaining of acute pains in the feet; blood tests revealed nothing, she was given pain killers and told to wear pure leather shoes. Further complaints of severe pain in her shoulder and difficulties in moving her arm were treated as torn ligaments. It was only after discharge from hospital following a hysterectomy that she went back to the practice still in pain, saw a different doctor and was referred for a specialist opinion. She reports being very annoyed when diagnosed as arthritic: 'I felt I'd gone six months without treatment, perhaps if I'd been treated in the early stages of it it might not have been so bad. In saying that I would also say that my doctor's marvellous, they've all been very good to me. But that doesn't alter the fact that I feel I went all those months without treatment and that was the starting of it.'

A minority of those interviewed experienced no delay between presentation and diagnosis, either because they consulted doctors who were familiar with the clinical picture of early rheumatoid arthritis, because onset was sudden or devastating or because the individual had delayed for so long that their situation was less ambiguous when they did present for medical attention. Mr S suffered onset while on leave from the army: 'It came on me straight away I just woke up stiff all over.' He was taken to hospital, diagnosed as having rheumatoid arthritis and within nine months had been discharged from the army 100 per cent disabled. Most, however, exhibited the classic picture of fluctuating and uncertain symptoms and fluctuating and uncertain interpretations, some of which were discarded and some of which were maintained over time until replaced by the formal diagnosis.

A medical diagnosis provides a solution to the cognitive problem posed by signs and symptoms; they are thereby legitimated and explained as the surface manifestations of an underlying pathological process. This is not the end of the matter, however, for once diagnosed persons with rheumatoid arthritis may be concerned with the question of why this has happened. They want to know the causes of rheumatoid arthritis in order that they may understand why they have acquired the disease. With diseases whose aetiology is not known, medical science cannot begin to answer this question, and patients are left to construct their own theories (Bury 1982). Some were only concerned with cause and searched their immediate pasts in the attempt to locate some factor which might be deemed responsible. Miss B had worked in a laundry and thought it might be caused by damp, and Mr M, who worked in a plastics factory, wondered if the chemical fumes had anything to do with it, 'because the factory inspector came round and done his nut about the amount of fumes in there'. He was so taken with this explanation that he wrote to the producers of a television programme he had seen on the occupational causes of disease who referred him to a specialist at a well-known hospital in London. Although the specialist dismissed his interpretation, a letter was sent to his consultant, and he felt he received more attention as a result: 'I've still got the feeling at the back of my mind that there may be something in it and no one's saying.' He was annoyed with his own doctor because, 'he never bothered to ask what I thought caused it'. Some searched their family history in order to locate other cases, and Mrs N ended up somewhat bewildered because her husband's mother had the disease, 'it's funny, it runs in his family but it's me that's got it'. When Mr I's doctor asked if he had ever worked in the mining industry, he decided it must be caused by dust in the joints, and Mrs X thought it 'might be to do with the sex organs' when a consultant pointed out that her major flare-ups had followed pregnancies and a hysterectomy.

Evident in some of the respondents' accounts was what Blaxter (1976:221) referred to as the strain towards rationality. This she defined as 'strenuous attempts to see their medical history as a whole, to connect everything that happened to them in the attempt to provide a coherent story in which effect followed cause in a rational way'. When asked to describe the onset of their condition, these people frequently started with childhood illnesses which were reinterpreted as rheumatic in nature and thought to be early warnings of the disease. Mrs R looked back and said 'I think I was having it when I was very young but didn't know what it was.' Her sister had suffered onset shortly after a fall, and Mrs R was able to remember a fall she had had when only 16. Mrs O connected onset to being knocked off her bicycle and Mrs K to her husband's coronaries. Not all tried to organize their life histories in this way or even to speculate about the nature and origins of the disorder. Like Mrs J who said 'I don't know what it is, I don't care, I've got it and that's it', these people appeared to be no longer troubled by the seemingly random hand of fate.

Problematic aspects of medical care

Given the difficulty of diagnosing and treating chronic illness, it might be expected that the long-term sick would be less satisfied with medical care than their non-impaired counterparts. Patients with rheumatoid arthritis might be expected to be particularly dissatisfied if only because there is no cure for the disease, available treatments are palliative and might not reduce pain or reduce it partially and for limited periods, many of the drugs used have exceptionally unpleasant side effects, and operative procedures are often painful and unsuccessful. Recent data concerning the views of disabled and non-disabled people partially supports this picture. Comparing the responses of the two groups to statements concerning general characteristics of doctors and statements about their own doctors, Patrick *et al.* (1982) report that non-disabled respondents were more dissatisfied with doctors in general while the disabled, particularly those whose disability was wholly or partially psycho-social, were more dissatisfied with their own doctors, especially with respect to personalized care. In this study no attempt was made to derive satisfaction scores or to evaluate medical care using consumer reports. Rather, in the course of the interviews patients were asked simple questions such as 'How often do you see your consultant/doctor?' 'When did you last see your doctor and what happened?' and were encouraged to talk about their experiences of medical care. If any general picture emerged at all, it was that the respondents tended to be more appreciative of doctors who were conspicuously concerned with their welfare and not just their medical condition and who were felt to have maintained an interest in their case. This seemed to hold irrespective of whether the doctors were successful in bringing about a marked improvement in their clinical condition. This can best be illustrated by examining those aspects of medical care which they found to be problematic.

In many respects the difficulties the chronic sick face in obtaining medical care are not too dissimilar from those experienced by patients in general. That is, all patients may encounter a variety of organizational and interactional barriers which must be negotiated en route to a satisfactory outcome (Locker 1981). Where these barriers are insurmountable, a deep disaffection may result, with the patient left feeling unimportant and abandoned by a service on which they are so dependent.

Access

The first problem disabled people face en route to medical care is that of access. Even though all were registered with general practitioners in the local community, many were so severely limited in their ability to walk that the physical effort involved in getting to the practice was a constraint on the frequency with which they would consult. The physical location of specialists in major hospitals around London made them even more remote so that a visit involved a major logistical exercise and often consumed an entire day. In an attempt to maintain continuity of care, some travelled considerable distances in order to see the doctor who had always dealt with their case, and this usually meant planning ahead to secure the necessary transport or spending considerable sums on hired cars. Until he changed to a hospital nearer home, Mr H had been spending £10 for a taxi to take him to the clinic and home again. Those with cars sometimes fared little better than those without. Mr F preferred to drive to the hospital, but limited space in the car park often meant that he could not persuade the attendant to let him in. On those occasions he was forced to find a parking space nearby, and this usually involved a walk that at best was painful and at worst beyond the limits of his tolerance. Because he had not applied for a disabled person car badge, illegal parking was costing him too much in fines, and he finally decided to use public transport.

Public transport is not and often cannot be designed with the needs of disabled people in mind. While buses may be built in ways which make getting on and off possible for those with limited strength and mobility, it is more difficult to ensure that bus stops and bus routes are conveniently situated and that long waits are avoided by buses running on time. Mrs J's main problem was having to stand to wait for buses. If she was lucky and was able to get a bus there and back fairly quickly, the journey to the hospital was manageable. At times she was standing for half an hour waiting for buses so that she arrived at the hospital in pain and arrived home thoroughly exhausted. Mr F found the journey by public transport so difficult that he wondered whether it was worth continuing to go to the hospital. When first interviewed he had been going weekly for heat treatment: 'It's very relaxing, it's beautiful while I'm there but then I've got to get up and get to the bus and I'm exhausted by the time I get there, back to where I started. I can't see what good it is pushing myself up there.' He found the journey to the hospital relatively manageable; the bus stop was near his home, and there was only a short walk at the other end when he got off the bus. The journey back was much more problematic. Getting to the bus stop meant negotiating busy roads and pedestrian underpasses, and where he got off the bus was not so conveniently situated for home, the local one-way system involving him in a much longer walk. To the person with limited mobility, an accumulation of such obstacles eventually defeats the purpose of the journey itself.

Mrs V was the oldest respondent and received little in the way of medical care. 'I can't get out for one thing, I'm transported wherever I go. Even my doctor . . . for my tablets I just have to get on the phone. I feel a fraud asking him to come out and I don't think they like coming anyway. So I get no treatment for the arthritis, nobody looks at it.'

Where hired cars and public transport were ruled out by the cost or effort involved, the people were forced to rely on the help of friends or transport provided by the hospital. Because it was necessary to fit in with the routines of the ambulance service, long waits at the hospital were unavoidable.

> *Mr I:* If you go up by ambulance you're sitting up there for three hours before your appointment . . . to me that's pointless, then you're not getting home again till half past seven at night. If you're appointment ain't till three and they come at twelve you've got to go.

Another feature of hospital organization which annoyed many respondents was the gap between the time they were told to arrive and the time they eventually saw the doctor. It was difficult for them to see any logic in this.

Mr M: I can never understand why they do that, why they say 9.30 and they don't see you till 12. Okay, so they're going to see so many each day, a half an hour per patient, fair enough, they know how long it's going to take to see me and most of the patients they should know how long it's going to take unless it's a new one and that can go at the end.

The physical difficulties involved in getting to the hospital and the long wait when they finally arrived became even more intolerable when the investment of time, energy, and money produced very little in the way of a return. Several felt that their visits to a specialist clinic were not very productive.

Mr I: All of a sudden you see him for two minutes, you've been in for two minutes, then I come back and say 'I've got to go and see my own doctor for me gold injection 'cus they wouldn't give it me there.' I get more sense out of me own doctor than what I was doing with that young doctor up there. I was only in there two minutes. He says 'Do you need any tablets, do you want a prescription, er, when's your gold due?' I might say 'Tomorrow.' 'Oh, go to your own doctor.'

Mr H and Mr M also felt that their visits were repetitive and pointless and produced very little in the way of a positive outcome.

Mr H: I'll sit there for a couple of hours and if I'm lucky I'll see the consultant and if I'm not I'll see the registrar and at the end of which he'll say 'Keep taking the Indecit and the aspirin and come back in three months.' Every time I go the registrar says what drugs are you on and every time they write down what drugs I'm on. If they read the damn file they'd find out for themselves, but there you are.

Mr M: They look at you, they turn this, they turn that and out you go. You don't come out cheered up or anything 'cus the same ruddy thing happens every time.

It is very likely that many of these visits for specialist attention were routine, and unless new symptoms had developed or side effects from drugs appeared, there was very little that could be done. If this is the case then the complaints documented above might be taken to be evidence of unrealistic expectations on the part of those concerned. Other data would suggest that this is not so; many realized that little could be done to improve their physical condition but looked to doctors for advice, information, and support. The length of time they were kept waiting, brief consultations, and the lack of any discussion of their problems were all interpreted as a lack of interest in their case. Mr E had not been impressed when his consultant told him not to come back for nine months so he changed to a hospital where he was seen every three, and Mr H had been very annoyed on a number of occasions when his consultant had not been available at his appointments, believing he gave priority to his students rather than the patients. After cancelling one appointment because of an ambulance strike, he had been waiting five weeks to be given another. All this he took to be indicative of an underlying attitude.

> *Mr H:* Now, is this man going to see me or not, because if he isn't then he's clearly and utterly indifferent. Now I know there's nothing he can do. I'm quite well aware of that fact, but it's this couldn't-care-less, don't-give-a-damn attitude. Everytime I go down there we sit for two hours and then see the registrar or the consultant comes along and says 'I'm sorry I can't see you, I've got to lecture to medical students.'

The amount of personal interest shown by the doctor also figured in Mr I's comparison of his general practitioner, original consultant, and the doctor he currently saw at the hospital.

> *Mr I:* I can sit there for ages talking to my doctor, he's really interested an' all, he'll sit there and listen you know, he says 'If there's anything in line for you I'll put you in for it, don't worry about that.' At the hospital, two minutes and you're out. The first doctor was a terrific guy, really good, you know. You'd go in there, he'd sit you down and talk with you for about twenty minutes, half an hour, and he know people's waiting outside but he didn't bother, you know, all the ins and outs, how have you been getting on during the week an all that. Everyone said 'Ain't it a shame he left?'

Many studies of patient satisfaction with medical care have revealed that the majority of patients are more concerned with the personal qualities of doctors than their clinical expertise (Cartwright 1964). In the context of chronic illness, where therapeutic intervention is rarely successful, the quality of the doctor-patient relationship is even more important to the patient's sense of well being. Indifference, whether real or perceived, not only creates hostility but also the feeling that the patients and their problems are of little significance. As Mrs H said of her husband's case at the end of the interviewing, 'I know there's nothing they can do but if they took an interest it would make such a difference.' These cases can be contrasted with that of Mrs W who had been seen by the same specialist for over fifteen years despite the fact that he did nothing other than give her repeat prescriptions: 'I'm still under them from all these years and they never say, which I am indeed very grateful for, "Go to your own doctor. Get your drugs off him." '

The communication of information

So much has been written about communication in medical practice that no extended discussion is necessary here. Many studies have been published which document the extent to which patients in general are dissatisfied with the amount of information they are given during consultations, and the chronic sick are no exception (Patrick *et al.* 1982). It could be argued that the communication of information is even more important with respect to chronic illness since the patient not only has to manage a variety of distressing symptoms but also has to learn to adapt to new and more limited life styles. Some would go as far as to claim that for many chronic illnesses the communication of information is the only form of treatment there is (Joyce *et al.* 1969). The general impression given by this small group of people is that they had been told relatively little other than the diagnosis, the fact that rheumatoid arthritis was incurable, and that rest was essential to prevent undue inflammation of the joints. If they had been given extensive advice on ways to manage the disease or reorganize their existence, then it had not been remembered.

There are a number of reasons why communication between doctors and their chronically sick patients may be or may appear to be poor. Blaxter (1976) cites organizational failures, misinterpretations by the patient, genuine clinical uncertainty, and the therapeutic management of information. It may also be due to doctors' operational ideologies concerning the management of patients (McIntosh 1974) and their images of patients and doctor-patient relationships from which decision rules about information giving are derived (Commarroff 1976). It is not possible to sort out from patients' accounts which of these reasons are responsible in individual cases; it is only possible to describe what aspects of information giving are problematic. It must be remembered, however, that not all the respondents were critical about how much they were told since not all desired more information than they were given. They varied from Mrs J who knew little about rheumatoid arthritis and did not feel it important that she did know, to Mr H, Mrs G, and Mrs L who wanted to know exactly what was happening, either because they valued information for its own sake or because it was necessary for them to organize an appropriate response. Mrs G said 'I must know in words of one syllable so I can understand, you can always make peace easier with something you can understand than something you don't.' She wanted information about her condition and her prognosis so she could plan in the long-term and in the short-term so she could do whatever was necessary to enhance her clinical status. She did not know whether to rest or to take exercise: 'I don't know where to begin, you see if they told me in words of one syllable I could adjust accordingly, but at the moment I'm completely in the dark.'

A common complaint among those who wanted information about their condition was the lack of any general discussion of their case and also the difficulty of getting a satisfactory reply to direct questions.

Mr M: No one has got hold of me and sat me down and given me a great deal of discussion, it's just been a matter of, 'Oh, you've got it', you know. It's very depressing actually 'cus no one is really giving answers to questions. I asked questions, why did they take blood tests? and things like that. They said that'd give quite a lot of answers but they weren't giving me the answers. In my job I had to give answers to questions and I expect the same thing from them. Maybe it's because I'm not asking the right questions.

Mr H: No one will tell you anything. You see, I turn this hand and you see it shakes. Now I say to the doctor, the Consultant, 'What causes this?' And he says 'Oh, you don't want to worry about that, it's nothing to worry about.' So you see, I can't find out what it is.

Another complaint was that doctors rarely revealed the reason for doing certain tests or the results when they were completed.

Mr M: I was up there three weeks ago and I complained about the pain in my back and he called a chap over and they said, 'We'll X-ray it but it won't show anything,' and I thought 'Well it's pointless them taking an X-ray if it won't show anything' and yet I was in considerable pain. I get the impression sometimes they think you're conning them, they don't believe that you're in the pain you're in. Either they don't believe you or the tests they're doing don't comply with what I've got. He never said 'Come back to see the result of that X-ray the same day or a fortnight's time.' I know the answer could be given the same day but I've got to wait three months for the result and I'm in agony. I never feel happy when I come out of there. I say to myself 'Well, that was a waste of time.'

Where doctors appear to be evasive or do not give patients the information and answers they seek, a variety of conclusions may be drawn. One is that the doctors are unsympathetic or uncaring, another that they have reached the limits of their expertise and do not know what to do, and yet another that they are concealing the truth about the patient's condition because it is too awful to reveal. Mr H and Mrs G were both severely disabled, had complicated conditions involving may symptom groups, and wanted but did not get acceptable responses to their many questions concerning prognosis. Given the lack of interest shown in his case, Mr H had his own ideas about his chances.

Mr H: It's quite obvious I'm branded as a write-off. Well, why not say so and be finished with it, you see. I mean, a lot of people don't like to be told these things, but I like to be told exactly where I am. If they say 'Look, boyo, your number's up, you'll be dead three months from now.' Fair enough, it doesn't bother me, but they don't, they just leave us.

Mrs G wanted a full and frank discussion of her problems simply because her situation was intolerable. She was blind, in severe pain, lived alone, and was rapidly being beaten by the struggle of day-to-day living. She felt that a great deal of damage had been done by interactions between the many drugs that had been prescribed and wanted this acknowledged so that the slate could be wiped clean, her condition reassessed, and a fresh start made. Her relationship with her doctors was clearly full of conflict, and she believed they neither listened to her complaints, accepted her suggestions as to what might be done, or even told her the truth. Her main problem, one which caused her a great deal of distress, was her lack of mobility, and she was convinced that hydro-therapy would get her legs going again:

> *Mrs G:* I keep getting answers which to me are less than honest. One said to me 'Well, of course it exercises the wrong muscles.' It's not true. Another said to me 'You can't have hydrotherapy on the National Health,' that's not true either. I wish to heaven if they have something to say tell me the truth, you know, I'm over 21, I'm my own next of kin, I'm all grown up. I *can* have the real answers. If not hydrotherapy then I want an honest answer. If the doctor has something to say, say it *to* me not *about* me. They're inclined to go into little huddles in a corner which I don't particularly like.

Given her difficulty in getting answers which she accepted as honest, Mrs G was convinced there was something amiss which was not being revealed; she believed their techniques for avoiding giving her informa-tion were designed to conceal past mistakes and a current uncertainty as to what to do.

> *Mrs G:* I come away with the impression why are they lying, if they're having to lie what is it they can't tell me? I think they got themselves into a terrible muddle over drugs, I think they've run out of know how, you see, they're probably up a gum tree.

Another aspect of communication which sometimes led to a loss of faith in doctors and medical care was the lack of consensus between different clinicians concerning diagnosis, treatment, and prognosis. This is almost inevitable in the case of chronic illness; many doctors are involved in the management of any patient, and the uncertainty surrounding the case provides plenty of opportunity for disagreements to arise. In fact, some respondents deliberately sought different opinions in the hope of finding a doctor who would offer a more favourable prognosis and course of action. Blaxter (1976) suggests that patients often misinterpret these differences, seeing them as evidence of the incompetence of some doctors and not as different parts of the truth about their condition seen from different clinical perspectives. In some cases this may be so; in others the patients' perceptions more nearly seem to reflect real conflicts of opinion between specialists. Because patients are often not made aware of uncertainty and the tentative nature of many medical judgements, discrepancies in what they are told lead them to doubt the skill of some who have had responsibility for their case. Mr H's recent history was full of such disagreements and discrepancies about diagnosis and appropriate procedure. His arthritis was complicated by a severe breathlessness that was as debilitating as the pain and malformation of his joints; he had been told by one doctor that it was emphysema and by another that it was connected to the arthritis and caused by an accumulation of fluid in the lungs. He had been subject to an exploratory knee operation at one hospital, following which he had rarely walked, only to be told at his current hospital that the operation had been unnecessary and the problem would have resolved itself in due course. A doctor from an emergency medical service he called during the night gave him an injection of what he was told was a heart stimulant; his GP, who came the next morning, said ' "That's the last thing you should have had." ' He was told by an orthopaedic surgeon at the hospital that nothing could be done to straighten his fingers, while a consultant he saw following his application for an electric wheelchair said an operation was possible, and he could only conclude 'Either they can't do anything or they're being indifferent, I don't know which.' Finally, he had been sent by his current consultant for exercise in the hospital hydrotherapy pool:

> *Mr H:* That nearly killed me. They stuck me in this hydrotherapy, like a swimming pool, you know, there's so much salt in it it's like the Dead Sea and it was as horrid as hell. It was humid you see and with this chest trouble I couldn't get my breath. So I'm gasping for breath and it took three of them youngsters to haul me out after about two minutes. And they said 'I can't understand the specialist putting him in here, we never have people with chest troubles in this pool. It's the last thing you should have been given.' We've got to the point where they all disagree amongst themselves. One says one thing and one another. You don't know what is right and which is wrong.

During the course of an illness career, patients may come to a number of conclusions about their needs for medical care. Television programmes about new operations or drugs, newspaper articles, and the accounts of fellow sufferers give them ideas about interventions which they believe will improve their condition and reduce levels of disability. Treatments they have received in the past may acquire favour and be seen to be worth another try. The problem then is to get their doctors to accept their point of view and proceed accordingly. This, of course, is a strategy fraught with danger; the doctor may interpret the patient's request as a reflection on his or her competence, and conversely, patients may take a refusal to comply with their request as a reflection on them. Different definitions of what is needed thus give rise to covert if not overt conflict, and patients may shop around for a doctor who will provide the treatment they think they need. For example, Mrs W changed hospitals and specialists when her doctor refused to refer her for a hip operation:

> *Mrs W:* You see, this woman had it done and she was walking about perfectly with a limp and I thought there's me lying around in bed half the time or crawling around and crying as though I wished I were dead so I thought I'd try that. I did ask the surgeon but he said 'No way will we do that. We'll treat you the best way.'

When first seen, Mr F had recently had joint operations on his right hand which had increased his manual dexterity to such an extent that he could now pick things up and manipulate small objects. Unfortunately, he had limited movement in his right shoulder and could not comb his hair or wash his back. The left hand was completely useless but the left arm fully mobile because the shoulder on that side was unaffected by arthritis. Mr F thought that further operations would restore his capacity to work, and though he had not suggested this to his doctors, he became very critical of the care he had received.

> *Mr F:* I was hoping they'd do more operations but as I say, I don't like to criticize the doctors but I think I'm wasting my time going down there. I went down home to Cornwall at Easter and there's two girls down there, down the road from where I live, and they've got exactly the same as I've got and they've had operations on their legs and hips, one's had their knees done and one their hands and that's just a cottage hospital compared to mine, so it makes me wonder why I've got to wait, I've been there 12 years now I suppose.
> *Int:* Have you talked about the possibility of an operation?
> *Mr F:* No, they haven't mentioned it at all. I have literally given up 'cus I can't understand how it could go on so long, I'm just going to wait now and get out of London completely.

Mr F had been to see a surgeon currently treating his mother-in-law and had been told that an operation would be feasible once he had moved and been discharged from the care of the doctors currently dealing with his case. He was very annoyed that nothing was being done, 'because I can't get about properly or anything', but was directing his energies to finding a house and possibly work in the country.

Other discrepancies in definitions of need gave rise to overt conflict between the respondents and their doctors. Sometimes this conflict paid off, as in the case of Mrs D who kept 'on and on' at her doctor until she was finally referred to a rehabilitation unit, but sometimes it did not. At the first interview, Mrs G was being treated by a specialist she labelled a physician and thought a rheumatologist or neurologist might be of some help. She was anxious to try hydrotherapy and planned to ask her doctor at the next appointment. Soon after the consultation she gave this account:

> *Mrs G:* There must be something in there that's rather derogatory, something that makes a doctor change his tone of voice, you know what I mean, 'cus I said 'How about the rheumatology department? How about the neurology department?' To which he leaned back in his chair and said 'This is a neurology department. This is a rheumatology department.' To which I would say 'Piffle!' I didn't but that's what I felt like saying 'cus it just isn't true. And I did say 'How about hydro-therapy?' and he said to me 'Well, where do you want to go to hydrotherapy? Lourdes?' Well, I am a believer but that wasn't quite what I had in mind, you know, he was just being sarcastic.

Patients' requests for treatments such as hydrotherapy are not derived solely from a belief that they will effect a dramatic improvement; while they may be of practical value, making the attempt is almost as important as the outcome.

> *Mrs G:* I don't know what to do, the only thing I would really like to have a shot at is hydrotherapy and I can't quite understand why it's turned down. I know from experience that if I get into warm water it does relieve pain and being buoyant would give mobility to the legs and if there's enough life in them to walk again it would prevent deterioration of the muscles. Whether they agree with me is another matter, but I think it would be helpful if only psychologically, I think I would feel something was being *done*. At least I would have thought it's worth a try.

From the patient's point of view, almost any intervention is better than nothing; even if they do not bring direct results, treatments are indicative of concern and are appreciated as such. Mr H made this point when he said:

> *Mr H:* One doesn't expect a miracle cure, but one does expect, shall I say, sympathetic interest. This hand is bending down more and more but they could at least put a splint on it, *try* and straighten it out, *try* and stop this one going the same way.

The experience of Mrs G and Mr H can be contrasted with that of Mrs A who spoke glowingly of her consultant: 'He's very helpful, he's willing to try anything and everything to give me some relief.'

An apparent unwillingness on the part of doctors to attempt operations or other therapeutic procedures may be part of the process whereby the chronically sick and disabled come to realize that as far as medical care is concerned, they are 'written off'. While many know and accept that nothing can be done, it is a different matter to be told this or to become aware of it when doctors appear to have abandoned the case or are not prepared to make a significant effort on their behalf. It is distressing to these people because it makes it difficult to maintain hope. It is even more distressing for those who will not accept that nothing can be done and believe they can fight their way back to some semblance of an active existence, because it means they are left to fight alone. Mrs T was a good example of the former. She had not received specialist attention for a number of years but decided to request a domiciliary visit when she had an acute flare-up which left her in a very bad way. The following extract is taken from an interview conducted soon after that visit.

> *Mrs T:* I do understand that a rheumatologist who's any rheumatologist has really only got to walk into a room and look at me and if the man knows his job he will know there's virutally nothing he can do to help me but I suppose that one likes to keep up pretences as far as one can and the fact that he only stayed ten minutes was a bit of a body blow to me. I thought to myself afterwards, 'Don't be stupid you knew before he came there was nothing he could do.' None the less it was a bit of a psychological blow.
>
> *Int:* What disappointed you about the fact he was here for such a short time?
>
> *Mrs T:* It was several things . . . I suppose it's all summed up in the phrase I felt I was written off. Now that is a stupid thing to feel and totally unjust to the consultant concerned because if I'm honest I knew I was written off before he came but I suppose the old business of hope springing eternal, even just the thought that there might be a straightforward pain killer, I think it was just the thought being brought to the forefront of my mind that I was written off, not in a nasty way, he wasn't in any way unsympathetic, he was a very pleasant and understanding man but after all if he'd stayed here for an hour and half the sum total of his visit would have been exactly the same. So to criticize him for the length of time he stayed is wrong but I did feel resentful . . . stupid and ridiculous, but I did none the less.

Mrs G refused to admit that nothing could be done and was determined to become sufficiently mobile to go back to her job as a teacher. She described herself as a fighter, and by her own efforts had often managed to salvage what appeared to be a desperate situation and return to a relatively active life. Unlike Mrs T, she was very critical of her medical care.

> *Mrs G:* I want to get better . . . I don't know whether that's pie in the sky but I'm certainly going to try and, you see, I really wish they

wouldn't give up on me, that again is psychologically bad if you feel the doctor's given up or even if he tells you so, which is worse. I think that's bad, they should work with you and not say 'Oh dear,' you know, or even say 'Sorry, we goofed but let's pick up the pieces that are still here.' I feel they are giving up on me, everybody. It's a little disheartening and one doctor came into me and said 'Well, of course, you're getting old,' and I said 'What? You've got to be kidding, I may look it but I'm not.' So he said 'You're not, your body is,' and so 'Well, thanks a bunch.' And he went off and I've since changed doctors. I must have a doctor who works with me. OK, so you don't know what to do, but you *can't* give up. I'm still here, much to everyone's surprise but I'm still here.

Mrs G was visited regularly by the Social Services Rehabilitation Officers and had been supplied with all manner of aids and appliances. While these helped her to manage at home, they had only a limited contribution to make towards the achievement of her major goal, controlling pain and getting mobile again. Consequently, she was dependent upon medical intervention: 'In practice everything has been done, meals on wheels, the wheelchair, grab rails, all the trappings are there but I'd like some help *in myself.*' Clearly, Mrs G had high expectations of herself and her doctors. Arguably, they were essential for her to maintain the hope of improvement and thereby prevent her 'giving up' and accepting the inevitability of residential care.

Other respondents felt, or had been told, that as they aged their case was no longer a priority, scarce resources being reserved for the young who offered a better return on the investment. Mr H reported being told ' "Well, of course, you are 60. If you were 25 we'd take much more interest in your case, we'd try to do very much more. After all at 60 two-thirds of your life is over." ' His initial reaction had been one of, 'Well, that's very comforting, isn't it?' but on reflection he was able to see a kind of logic in it. As could those who thought they were 'too far gone'; why take up the doctor's time when there were other people who he could help? Mrs R rather regretted that kind of attitude for no matter how justified, it seemed to mean that new and distressing symptoms were not taken seriously, properly investigated and treated.

> *Mrs R:* I've always had very good treatment wherever I've been, it's only now I've got older, and I think this is what is rather a shame, you get brushed off. As you get older I think you're inclined to get brushed off. You see, I'm having terrific trouble with my eyes and I know that if I could get my eyes right I could get going again, but I think they've put it down to arthritis, you know, 'You've got arthritis' and that's it. When you're young you get away with an awful lot, you get made rather a fuss of but when you get to my age you're brushed off.

Mrs R's eyes were sore and inflamed; she found it difficult to drive and was embarrassed because they watered frequently, so much so that she had stopped going out if it was necessary to meet other people. She said she had mentioned it to the doctor 'over and over again' and thought of going privately for treatment. She had been given a letter to take to the hospital but having already been there was not confident that anything would be done. Her daughter said: 'It's the same attitude, it's the same if you go to the hospital, you see a different doctor, one look at the wheelchair and that's it, you know, "You've got arthritis. This won't bother you much, so carry on." '

Not all respondents encountered these kinds of problems in their dealings with the medical profession; some doctors, predominantly GPs, were very highly regarded because they showed the sympathetic interest desired, were very helpful with regard to benefits and other services, and were willing to acquiesce to the patient's request for new drugs or alternative forms of treatment. As Mr H said 'It's a matter of finding yourself a good chap.' Where doctors are perceived to be reluctant to give information or modify their treatment plan in accordance with the patient's wishes, there is very little the patient can do. Because doctors control the cognitive and material resources necessary to solve the patient's problems and also the course of the consultation itself, patients may have very little opportunity to exert an influence on medical decision making. They may attempt to persuade or bargain, or they may conceal information from the doctor to avoid courses of action they view as undesirable. Mr P had not mentioned his depression to his doctor, fearing that he might be pressured into accepting residential care, and Mrs R initially concealed a rash produced by gold injections because she did not want the drug, believed to lead to a cure, to be withdrawn. Where these tactics fail the patient has little option but to grudgingly accept the doctor's opinion or seek help elsewhere. The chronically sick and disabled person may then be left struggling to maintain the hope of a better future in the light of the knowledge that nothing is being or can be done.

Therapeutic intervention

The therapeutic measures available to treat rheumatoid arthritis fall into three categories: drugs, operations, and various forms of physiotherapy. The main drugs employed are aspirin, nonsteroidal anti-inflammatory drugs, gold salts, Penecillamine, and cortico-steroids. Operative procedures range from the aspiration of fluid from inflamed joints to surgical immobilization or total replacement of affected joints, and physiotherapeutic procedures may involve controlled exercise, heat treatment, and hydrotherapy. None of the drugs currently used are totally effective in eliminating inflammation and pain, and their impact may vary from patient to patient, so much so that many are subject to a trial-and-error procedure in which alternative drugs and dosages are prescribed to determine which is the best in the individual case. Moreover, all the drugs in use give rise to adverse reactions, and unpleasant side effects may be common. The operations on affected joints are usually exceedingly painful, requiring long periods of immobilization in plaster. To judge by the recipients' accounts, they are often unsuccessful, leaving the patient more limited than prior to surgical intervention. For the person with rheumatoid arthritis, all treatments involve a degree of risk, and the disadvantages may outweigh the advantages to be gained. As Mrs R said, 'It's not the disease that kills you, it's the treatment', a view supported by professional opinion (Hughes 1979).

The uncertainty that is characteristic of the disease also applies to the outcome of available treatments so that doctors and patients are frequently forced into situations of choice. As is almost always the case in the context of chronic illness, the advantages and disadvantages of any course of action must be carefully weighed in making decisions as to how to proceed. Doctors and patients may, of course, attach different values to these advantages and disadvantages to produce conflict: to Mrs G, hydrotherapy was worth a try, to her doctors it may have offered so little in the way of a return that it constituted nothing more than a waste of scarce resources. While the uncertainty surrounding therapeutic intervention could result in conflict, it also often led to co-operation; some respondents reported that their doctors did discuss the pros and cons of drugs and operations and in many instances left the final choice to them. There were, however, occasions when the respondents felt they had not been fully informed about the side effects of some drugs and what was involved in various operations or exploratory procedures. This gave rise to a great deal of resentment, particularly when the outcome was less than satisfactory.

As Strauss (1975) has discussed at length, therapeutic interventions take the form of regimens that have to be managed within the context of the person's everyday life. Conflicts may arise between the demands of the regimen and other social obligations which mean that one or the other or both may have to be modified. For example, Mrs Q and Mrs X reported that they had often discharged themselves from hospital earlier than advised because they were unhappy with the arrangements for the care of their children. Mrs R went so far as to wonder whether she might have been in a better state had her treatment not been continuously interrupted by the demands of motherhood. In this and other ways, adhering to medically prescribed regimens may cause as much trouble as the symptoms themselves. With some conditions the regimen is such that the person has little choice but to comply no matter how disruptive it proves to be. Dialysis patients, for example, have little room for manoeuvre and little opportunity for modifying the treatment in ways that make it more compatible with daily living. With diseases like rheumatoid arthritis there is choice, and regimens may be modified or adapted to bring them more in line with the individual's own goals and values. Consequently, patients are not totally powerless within the framework of medical care; once outside the surgery or clinic they are left to their own devices and can acquire a modicum of responsibility for their condition and its management.

Problematic aspects of therapeutic intervention

One problem chronically sick people encounter in the face of medical intervention is deciding whether to proceed with a drug or operation recommended by their medical advisers, family, or fellow sufferers. Drugs usually present less of a problem; they may be tried, and if found to be ineffective or to give rise to intolerable side effects, they can be discontinued. Even so, this trial-and-error approach may create a great deal in the way of discomfort and distress, particularly if several drugs are tried in turn and the individual must tolerate weeks of nausea, dizziness, and diarrhoea, only to find that aspirin was the most effective way of controlling pain in his or her case. When Mrs T was seen by a consultant during her acute flare-up, he suggested she try a number of drugs which had given good results to determine which was the best in reducing her pain.

> *Mrs T:* Anyway, the first one I tried resulted in a fortnight's very violent diarrhoea and to have to get up from bed five or six times a night when I was in dire distress with a bad knee wasn't funny so I'm afraid after that I chickened out and said 'No more, I'll just go back to aspirin.'

Where the side effects of a drug are known but there is no certainty that they will appear, individuals may decide to proceed in the hope that in their case the advantages will outweigh the disadvantages, and even if this is not so, it will become clear fairly quickly. In some instances the patient may have to decide to proceed with a drug that is so new that its side effects have not been documented. The risks then are much greater; even if side effects do not appear in the short term, there is no guarantee that irreversible damage will not be done over time. Nevertheless, Mrs W decided to go ahead and take a new drug designed to control the symptoms of a stomach ulcer caused by long-term aspirin and steroid therapy because it meant she could eat anything without discomfort: 'But what the side effects are . . . on that (laughs) I wouldn't know and neither do they yet. They can't say definitely none 'cus it's not been out long enough.' This woman had been on high dosages of steroids for many years and though these had been withdrawn had to continue on low dosages for the rest of her life to compensate for the atrophy of her adrenal glands.

Where the benefits and drawbacks of a drug are certain, patients and their doctors are in a better position to make a decision regarding their use. Steroids were avoided by many of the respondents because the gain in weight that followed seemed less desirable than pain. Mrs N, however, was forced to resort to steroid therapy because no other drug reduced the pain, and Mrs R accepted the necessity of injections of steroids when she reached an age at which her appearance was no longer of primary importance.

> *Mrs R:* You see, I've always been very thin and I was in hospital once and I overheard, you shouldn't listen to other people's conversations, but I overheard the nurses say 'Isn't it a shame? She's had these injections. She hasn't got the pain but she's got so fat she can't walk.' And this is what's happened to me. But for me it's a choice between the freedom from pain or the moon face and the effect the injections have. Well, my days of vanity are gone. If I was young well I wouldn't have cortisone but when you get older you don't care you just want relief from pain and that's that.

Mrs R kept on a low dose and tried to limit the injections to one a week in an attempt to minimize the side effects. By the time of the last interview, however, she had become concerned about her weight problem. Following a domestic dispute her daughter had left home, and she had spent two days in residential care. When it was time for her to return home the ambulance men refused to take her because she was so heavy, and she was forced to wait until two more could be found to assist them: 'I felt so stupid, I didn't think I was that big, you know, it's made me think. I'm trying to get off the injections because the weight problem is absolutely unbelievable.' Such an assault on her identity had clearly modified the values Mrs R attached to the various outcomes of this particular therapy so that she decided to try to abandon it altogether.

Deciding to go ahead with an operation is a more difficult matter; the outcome is often uncertain and once done surgery is irreversible. Over half of this group of people had had some form of operation on affected joints, and while many were successful in reducing pain and improving mobility, some were not, leaving the joint locked and virtually useless. To judge by their accounts, many of the respondents were more favourably disposed towards operations than their doctors, particularly if surgery had brought about some improvement in one of their joints, and some requested further attempts to restore the others. Some of these requests met with a refusal; surgery was insufficiently advanced to be of use in their cases. In others, the doctor advised against an operation, often because there was a degree of movement in the joint, but the chances of securing an improvement were such that they agreed to go ahead if the patient so wished. Mrs O was taken into hospital when she requested a knee operation she heard about via a radio programme and was advised not to go ahead since she was managing so well. The final decision was left to her, and when she discovered two other patients in hospital who had not been helped by the operation, she agreed with the doctor's assessment and was discharged. Decisions such as this required a careful balancing of risks and benefits. Where the limitations imposed by an arthritic joint were intolerable, then the individual often wanted to go ahead even though the chances of success were small. Then they eagerly recounted the experiences of those who had been helped by surgery in order to maintain their definition of an operation as being worth a try.

It is not only the risks involved that need to be taken into account when considering surgery, for the operation itself may be very painful and very disruptive of everyday life. Even where an operation is successful, a second may be delayed because of the discomfort it caused. Mrs W had been unable to hold or grip small objects until an operation to stiffen her thumb restored her capacity to pick things up. Despite the fact that 'it was a marvellous operation', it was four years before she could bring herself to have the other one done.

> *Mrs W:* I was so frightened because it's a painful operation. They do the joint a little, you can see where the surgeon cuts it through, but you've got to have your arm up in the air and the pain is absolutely terrific especially when you've got other bad joints. I was a bit of a coward and thought I wouldn't have this one done but it got so I couldn't pick anything up without dropping it so I decided I would. You're in plaster for three months, you feel at the time that you're never going to move your thumb again, the pain is terrific, it's afterwards it's wonderful.

It is not only operations which are unpleasant and painful; the other procedures used for managing rheumatoid arthritis may be equally so. Fluid is often drained from inflamed and swollen joints, and anti-inflammatory agents may be injected directly into the joint cavity itself. Consequently, some pain and discomfort may have to be tolerated in order to secure relief. These procedures can sometimes be so traumatic that the patient refuses to have them again.

> *Mrs J:* The first time I went to see Dr Y when I had this shoulder with the terrible, terrible burning agony, the very first time he injected into the joint and I've never had anything so revolting in all my life. And I come out of the hospital and I never went back to him again. I didn't

like that hospital, having had one daughter in there and found the place a filthy revolting hole I vowed and declared I'd never go back again and I didn't.

It was another four years before Mrs J, under pressure from her family, went to the hospital again and was immediately admitted for 11 weeks bed rest. Since then fluid had been drained from her knees a number of times, and she had developed a number of techniques for making the experience more tolerable.

Mrs J: When I had my shoulder done it was terrible it really made me feel ill. When I thought I was going to have me knees done I thought 'O God,' and every time I saw Dr C walk through them doors I felt sick wondering what was coming and then when he had done them the relief, it's worth two minutes of discomfort with the needles to have that relief from the fluid and the pain. Dr Y is marvellous, he just shifts me knee cap over and gives me this tiny injection and that's it. Because having the fluid off is very uncomfortable. It really is unless you get somebody who is a good needle man and knows what they are doing. Because to have the fluid drained off and the other stuff put in, well that is the worst part because it's so thick it has a bit of a job going in. But as I say if you get a good needle man that's all right. The first time I didn't know what to expect but I had a marvellous doctor do it, it was the registrar Dr C, he just froze my knee, sprayed, froze, injected, done, all over.

When a good needle man was not available, Mrs J would attempt to exercise her right of veto and refuse to have it done.

Mrs J: They asked me would I go to a doctors' seminar and let them watch, so I agreed, I agree to anything. When I got down there and I saw Dr S I said 'He's not doing it. Providing Dr C does it, fair enough.' I mean, Dr S was a very nice person but I had never had him give me injections, I like the tried and trusted I'm not a lover of strangers. Well, Dr C was elsewhere in the hospital so they had to bleep him and we had to wait. I kept the seminar waiting nearly an hour and he just got back to do my knees when he was called away on an emergency. So Dr S done them after all and it wasn't a very nice trip, I wasn't amused.

Another technique Mrs J used to cope with unpleasant therapeutic procedures was to give herself time to get used to the idea of having the procedure done. She described how her brother, also an arthritic, had been up to the hospital where he was offered an injection into his temperomandibular joint. He refused: 'I can understand it because he's had 13 operations he's really been through it. Even with myself, you've got to get accustomed to the idea of having this done. He's like me, you can't spring that sort of thing, you've got to accustom yourself.' Consequently, she always waited two or three weeks when fluid began to accumulate on her knees before having it taken off. The delay meant she could get used to the idea of having it done and, by then, the pain of the procedure was nothing compared to the pain of the swollen joint.

If chronically sick and disabled persons wish to take advantage of the potential benefits of surgical and other interventions, they have little choice but to tolerate the discomfort of operations and the inconvenience of long spells in hospital. Other aspects of their regimens, drugs, rest, and exercise, can be changed according to their own needs and daily routines. Many of the respondents modified the dosages of their drugs, taking more when in pain and less when the pain was not too severe. This allowed them to pursue what were often contradictory goals; achieving maximum relief from pain while minimizing the side effects and their dependency upon analgesics or anti-inflammatory preparations. Some used them sparingly or intermittently in the belief that 'when they've got used to me they won't act' or did not take them at all; Mr C: 'They only take the pain away for a few minutes and then it'll come back again so there's no use taking drugs if it's going to come back again so I never bother.' When the arthritis seemed to be quiescent and pain levels manageable, some tried to reduce their dosage drastically or do without the drugs altogether only to have their dependence reaffirmed: Mr I cut his dosage by half and then had to double the dosage to cope with the pain and swelling that followed. Mrs N went away for the weekend and accidentally left her tablets at home. Thinking that it might not matter, she did not go back to get them. The next morning she was in such pain the weekend was abandoned and she returned home to her drugs.

The chronically sick person's ability to develop a regimen which suits his or her needs was not always respected by health professionals who sometimes interfered or forced him or her to change. Mr M had been through a very trying period in search of a drug to control his pain and finally found one which he was able to use to his satisfaction. At one clinic appointment he saw a different doctor who insisted on a change of drugs, 'so I'm now back where I started'. Mrs R did not have steroid injections weekly as prescribed but spaced them according to her levels of pain. When her daughter went on holiday, she was visited by the district nurse who assisted with personal care and gave her the injections:

Mrs R: When she came I said 'I don't want an injection this week I haven't had much pain' and she said 'Oh no, we've got to give it to you, you're down for the injection, you must have it.' So I rang my doctor and he said 'No, don't have it if you don't want to.' Then I had a fall and was in a lot of pain so I asked the nurse for an injection and she said 'You can't, you're not down for it.'

People in general seem to be more concerned with the personal qualities of their doctors than with their technical competence, and data presented earlier suggests that chronically sick people also value personalized care. The apparent failure of diagnostic and therapeutic skills to figure highly in patient evaluations might come about because it is not an issue; many of the conditions taken for medical attention are self-limiting and would have got better without professional intervention. This is not the case with the long-term sick who are dependent upon such skills for improving or containing their disease. Consequently, prescribed regimens are evaluated for their efficiency in meeting this goal and so are the people who recommend them (Strauss 1975). If medical intervention does not bring about an improvement in the patient's condition, or if they are seen to result in further damage, then the competence of the doctor may be questioned. In addition, since the chronically sick person may be subject to the same procedure by many different people, he or she has the opportunity to compare the performance of one with the others. For example, Mrs J had a blood test every month which, incidentally, she loathed so much she reduced her doctor to hysterics by requesting that a blood sample be taken under a general anaesthetic.

> *Mrs J:* There again, get a good needle person and no problem. You get some who starts digging and poking about. I mean I can have my blood test and not a mark on me and the tenth one they'll leave a bruise like that. If I can have nine blood tests without leaving a mark why should the tenth one mark? That turns me right off.

Because the drugs prescribed for rheumatoid arthritis rarely give complete relief from pain, some of the respondents found it difficult to say categorically whether or not they were a help. The fluctuating character of the pain rendered their judgments tentative; during quiescent phases they would say the drugs seemed to be having an effect, only to have that opinion challenged by a bad spell or acute flare-up. The outcome of operations was somewhat easier to assess in terms of reduction of pain and improved mobility although sometimes one had to be sacrificed in order to gain the other. Mrs D had an operation on her elbow which meant she had no pain but a joint that was permanently fixed. She had been under age at the time of the operation and though the consequences may have been explained to her parents, she had not been forewarned and now wished it had never been done. Others had been helped enormously by surgical intervention, and some believed that their disabilities had been increased by what had been done to them. The latter would support their interpretation of events by stories which cast doubt on the competence of those who had been responsible for their care. For example, Mr H was subject to an exploratory knee operation and said he had not been able to walk since.

Mr H: They said 'We must operate on the knee.' So I said 'All right.' I discover that I get to the theatre under local anaesthetic, that didn't bother me, but I discover the young registrar is doing the operation. So I said 'Surely this should be an orthopaedic surgeon's job?' 'Oh no, that's not necessary.' So he goes to work you see and he gets on a little and I heard him turn to the theatre sister and say 'My God, there's a terrific amount of blood here' and 'Stop this lot.' She said 'Well, use a diathermy needle, that'll stop it.' He says 'What's that?' She says 'It's this thing here.' 'Oh, how do you use that?' She says 'You just clamp it on the blood vessel and it will seal it off.' So he says 'You show me.' So she clamps it on and up goes a puff of blue smoke and seals off the blood vessel. 'Oh,' he says 'that's a wonderful thing, I've never seen one of those.' Well, I thought, here I am lying on this table with my arteries sliced open and this clown says 'I've never seen one of these. How do you use this?' Well, honestly, it leaves you speechless!

Because of the limited effectiveness of prescribed regimens, two of the respondents developed their own methods of management or sought help outside the formal system of medical care. Mrs N had seen a television programme concerning the effects of diet on the progress of disease and thought there was no harm in giving it a try. Since then she had not eaten red meat, fruit, or anything she believed to contain a lot of acid. She learned to do without foods she had previously enjoyed and thought that a combination of drugs and careful eating had kept her arthritis under control. She had also been on a pilgrimage to Lourdes and was so convinced she was going to be well stopped taking her medication, only to be forced back to it by pain. Mrs K went every two weeks to a private physiotherapist who had taught Mr K how to manipulate his wife's joints. Mrs K had not been given physiotherapy at the hospital so that when they were told about this woman by a friend, they decided to pay for the treatment themselves. Mr K thought that he had been able to improve the condition of his wife's hands by manipulation and was now trying to do the same for her arms: 'I think it helps but obviously, it can't do any harm can it?' The woman was also a spiritual healer, and the K's had derived great comfort and peace as a result of her help and the spiritual guidance they received through her. As Mrs K concluded, 'There's a great deal more to this life than the body we walk around in.'

4 Practical problems
of everyday life

To the non-disabled person many, if not all, of the activities of daily living
are non-problematic; they are simply taken for granted, performed with
hardly any awareness that they are being performed at all. This contrasts
vividly with the experience of people disabled in some way. To them
some, and frequently all, activities of everyday life are a problem and
continually challenge energy, ingenuity, and character. For the person
disabled by rheumatoid arthritis, waking life is characterized by pain and
a constant striving to overcome the innumerable difficulties encountered
during the course of the day. At first glance, few of these problems appear
to be major ones; nevertheless, they can have a significant impact on life
chances. As Mrs G said, 'It's the little things where you come unstuck',
and Mr H commented 'It's the really simple things that beat you and this
is what is so frustrating about the damn thing.' There may only be one or
two steps, but for the person confined to a wheelchair, they can be an
insurmountable barrier and prevent access to desirable activities or
settings. Even when of little significance individually, an accumulation of
such problems can be devastating. When Mr P was asked to identify his
biggest problem he said 'It's just a collection of small things.' Consequently, getting through the day becomes an achievement in itself and usually
all that available time and energy will allow.

The way in which the character of everyday activities is transformed by
a disease such as rheumatoid arthritis can be illustrated by considering a
simple task like making a cup of tea. If hips and knees are affected so as to
make standing and walking difficult, and if hands and wrists are affected
so as to make carrying, holding, and gripping almost impossible, then
some or all of the following may be a problem: getting out of a chair,
walking to the kitchen, reaching into cupboards where materials and
utensils have inadvertently been put, lifting a bottle of milk from the
refrigerator, turning on a tap, holding the kettle while it is filled, lighting
the gas stove, pouring boiling water, carrying the tea back into the sitting
room. Clearly, if many of these individual activities are a problem, the
person will have to employ a variety of strategies in order to cope. These
include learning how to manoeuvre out of a chair, altering the immediate
environment in such a way that progress from room to room is

unimpeded but potentially supported, arranging for necessary materials to be kept on hand or arranging for a filled kettle to be left on the stove or using special aids and appliances to make some of the steps more manageable. Even so, all of the tasks involved in the activity may need to be performed slowly, carefully, and with forethought in order to reduce pain and minimize danger. The only alternative is to do away with the problem by doing without.

Whether or not a particular activity is problematic depends to a certain extent upon the nature of the context in which it is to be performed. Going to the toilet is no problem for those confined to a wheelchair if facilities are accessible, sensitively planned, and necessary aids and appliances available. Where the physical or social environment is not so favourable, toileting may become a major problem and an important barrier to occupational or recreational opportunities. Mrs W, commenting on the facilities in the building which housed the Social Services Department said, 'I'd never be able to work there. They'd have to push me down the road to the public convenience. Very nice that.' Similarly, the strategy employed to cope with a problem should it arise may also vary according to context and environmental circumstance. Mrs A had very little strength in her hands and wrists and found it very difficult to cut certain types of food. This was not always a problem, for when eating or entertaining at home or when out at a restaurant, she could exercise a degree of control to ensure that what was served was manageable. There was often no problem when she was out to dinner with close friends; she had made them aware of her difficulty, and they selected their menus accordingly. There were occasions, however, when at the home of friends or out at official functions, she had been given food she could not cut. If her husband was present, she would surreptitiously ask him to cut the food for her; if not, she refused things even though it caused offence rather than embarrass herself and others by struggling to manage the meal or asking for help.

While disabled people do acquire a range of strategies which enable them to avoid or cope with problematic aspects of daily living, they may be forced to adapt or extend their repertoire according to changing circumstance. Familiar problems may arise in unfamiliar settings, or settings where necessary resources are not available, so that strategies have to be designed and implemented rapidly. Alternatively, new problems may be encountered in familiar environments like the home; they may be unexpected so that the individual is suddenly at a loss how to cope. When Mrs N knelt down to clean her oven, she found she could not get up again (see Chapter 2) and was still thinking it through when someone came home to rescue her. Over time the person comes to think ahead, to anticipate problems, and to appreciate the fact that ordinary activities need to be meticulously planned. 'Thinking it out' becomes the order of the day.

The kinds of practical problems experienced by people with rheumatoid arthritis are, of course, a function of the severity of the disorder, the location of affected joints and the extent of residual damage to the joints themselves. For some, the problems of daily living varied according to the day-to-day fluctuation in their condition, some days being trouble free, others a total disaster. For the remainder, their arthritis had inflicted such damage that every day consisted of a succession of problems which had to be managed irrespective of levels of pain. Those confined to wheelchairs or bed all fell into this category as did those in the midst of an acute flare-up. For them all aspects of everyday life presented difficulty; sleeping, personal care, cleaning and shopping, and mobility around the community all had to be managed as best they could. For some of the people interviewed, solving problems of this kind became the limits of their world.

Sleep and rest

Few of those interviewed experienced no problem with sleep and rest so that the minority who were not woken during the night spoke of how lucky they were in escaping being disturbed. The majority, however, slept badly so that when Mrs V said 'I don't know what a night's sleep is', she might well have been speaking for them all. The main problem, of course, was pain. Pain made it difficult to achieve a degree of comfort sufficient for sleep to be possible in the first place or caused them to wake several times during the night. Mrs K was usually still awake at three in the morning, and Mr P rarely had a good night's sleep.

> *Mr P:* I just can't sleep through the night. This is my worst problem is sleeping. I get over on one side to go to sleep and I may get an hour and that hip and leg they start paining. I turn over and that starts giving me it and then the weight of the blankets on that one so that starts to hurt and eventually I'm only doing about half an hour, a quarter of an hour's sleep each time I turn.
>
> *Int:* Is it like that most nights?
>
> *Mr P:* Most nights yes, unless I'm really. . . . If I go about three to four days without proper sleep I do drop off and the night I've had a good sleep I feel quite all right.

Many of those who had a problem in sleeping disliked taking sleeping tablets, and some would avoid taking them even when the pain was very bad. Part of the reason was a fear of becoming dependent on yet another drug, partly because the heavy sleep they induced meant stiffness on waking, and partly because they had developed other ways of coping with an inability to sleep. Mrs V avoided sleeping during the day in case it affected her at night, and Mrs W would not stay in bed if she could not sleep.

Mrs W: I don't believe in sleeping tablets at all and wouldn't take them on any account. I don't sleep very well at all but if I go to bed and can't sleep I'll get up again and it doesn't hurt you because you do sleep eventually sometime or other, I think its a load of rubbish, sleeping tablets. If you do take them you wake up and you can't move you get so stiff. I like to have a clear head and just be myself. So I don't lay in bed, I'd sooner be up in the wheelchair going around.

Restlessness at night, especially where it involved getting in and out of bed several times, frequently gave rise to a change in the sleeping arrangements of the respondents and their spouses. In an effort to minimize the disruption to others, double beds would be changed to singles or where a separate bedroom was available the two would sleep totally apart. This was usually the case when the spouse worked and needed a good night's sleep. Mr S and his wife had separate bedrooms for a number of years before being forced to leave their flat by noisy and aggressive neighbours. They currently shared a room, and Mrs S had no option but to tolerate her husband's 'tossing and turning and being up half the night'. They were waiting to be rehoused and had been promised accommodation with enough space for each to have his and her own room. The F's did not have a spare room, and Mr F would often sleep on the settee downstairs rather than keep on waking his working wife. In this way the persons concerned attempted to limit the extent to which their problems impinged on others.

Where a person needs help to get in and out of bed, then others have to be disturbed in order to provide the necessary assistance. Mrs R sometimes had to wake her daughter if she needed anything during the night, and this sometimes led to friction: 'The last time I wanted her in the night I'd been shouting and calling and shouting and when she goes to sleep she goes to sleep, believe me. We've had bells fitted over the bed and everything. Now I've got a stick I try not to disturb her, I hate disturbing her at night.' Similarly, Mrs W could get out of bed unaided but had to wake her husband to help her back in.

Mrs W: He says I'm a damn nuisance because I'll stop up half the night and I'll get up, I will. I'll lay there and I'll think 'I'm hungry, I can't stay here, I'll get up,' and, of course, I read for hours and I think 'No, I'll get up I can't sleep.' He doesn't hear me because he goes off he snores his head off, and then I'll put the fire on, I might make a cup of tea and I'll think 'Oh hell, I wish this pain would go.' And perhaps I'll try and go back to bed without help and then I've got to wake him up to get my feet in. He says 'What's the time?' I say 'It's half past four.' He'll say 'Whatever have you been doing?' and I say 'Going around. I can't sleep.' So I like really to go to bed when I like, sort of thing.

Although the H's lived in a three-bedroom flat, Mrs H refused to move into another room; if her husband was awake during the night, she wanted to be awake too, even though he did not necessarily need help. If he was in need she did not want him to ring the bell to summon a nurse from the Nursing Unit downstairs but preferred to give him the care he required, calling on the nurses only as a last resort.

> *Mr H:* If I'm up, she's got to be at my side. She says 'Once you're in your grave I'll have all the time in the world and if you're up gasping for breath I'm going to be there.' So those two bedrooms are empty. She's an extremely loyal kid, extremely loyal, which is a godsend to me.

Ambulation and body transfer

Moving about is almost always a problem for people with rheumatoid arthritis. While they may retain the ability to walk, pain, stiffness, and lack of strength make for difficulty in transferring their body from one position to another. Getting in and out of chairs, getting in and out of the bath, and getting in and out of bed are difficult because they no longer have the capacity to support their body weight and manoeuvre at the same time. Even turning over in bed may be impossible without the use of some kind of aid. Unlike the paraplegic, the person with rheumatoid arthritis cannot develop one part of the body to compensate for a lack of strength in another, for the chances are that one or more joints in all the limbs will be affected. Consequently, they must rely on special techniques, aids, both supplied and improvised, and the help of others.

Ambulation problems begin immediately on waking; in fact, the early morning is often the most difficult time for many arthritic people. So much so that Mrs W said 'I hate the mornings when I wake up because it's a nuisance to get out of bed and get into the chair and until you can get circulated around a bit it isn't very good.' The difficulty arises because hours of immobility in bed mean that the joints are very stiff and have little movement so that any activity can only be performed very slowly. Some mornings it took Mrs A 'an age' to get from her bed to the bathroom, and she needed to get up early in order to be sure of being ready for work. Mr F always spent a half hour exercising in bed before he even attempted to get up. Only by moving about, rolling around, and stretching his limbs could he achieve a degree of movement in his joints sufficient for him to get out of bed. Even so, transferring from a lying position to a standing position required a special technique. He had learned how to twist his body in bed so that he could manually lower his legs to the floor; swift movements had to be avoided for they resulted in pain. He used the bedside table to pull himself to a standing position and once up was ready to face the next problem: 'Once I'm standing I'm usually pretty fair, as long as I can keep my balance, I've got to have nothing in front of me.' Getting into bed required a similar procedure; he had to lift his right leg in manually, and after swinging his body in after it, he used his left leg to push the right one straight.

The difficulty the respondents faced in getting in and out of bed cannot be exaggerated. Low beds were a particular problem. For Mrs A 'it's just a case of rolling and manoeuvring until one gets into bed . . . it is a bit painful', and before Mr P swapped his low bed for a hospital bed, getting out took almost an hour of continual effort. Mr I could not get out of his low bed without the help of his wife so it was raised on castors and finally exchanged for a high orthopaedic bed. In spite of having a specially high bed, some still had difficulty achieving a standing position and had to break the manoeuvre down into stages with periods of rest in between.

In all, four of the respondents needed help to get into or out of bed, three of whom were confined to a wheelchair. Mr H and Mrs R were dependent upon hoists which could only be used with the assistance of others, while Mrs W could get out of bed but needed to be helped in. She had been provided with a hoist to use in the bathroom and bedroom in an attempt to make her more independent and less reliant upon her husband. Unfortunately, the ceiling fitting in the bedroom was inconveniently placed, and there was no way Mrs W could transfer the heavy lifting mechanism from one room to another by herself. Consequently, the hoist was kept permanently in the bathroom, and she continued to need help. While she was able to support herself on the bedside table to twist her body from the chair to the bed, her legs still had to be lifted in after her: 'So if I was on my own I'd just have to sit up all night.' She had developed a 'special way' of getting out of bed; by leaning in a particular direction and enlisting the forces of gravity to move her legs, she could manage alone. Mrs V also needed help to get her legs into bed. She initially relied on her husband, 'that was his job', but since his death had been left to struggle with just the help of a pulley over the bed: 'Now I'm on my own it makes life so difficult.'

Mr H's main problem with body transfer was a lack of strength in his limbs and an inability to grip. He could no longer hold a razor firmly enough to shave and had difficulty lifting a cup of tea. He spent all of his time in bed or in his wheelchair, and even with the help of the hoist, it was almost impossible for him to be placed anywhere else.

Mrs H: You see the problem is to get him from this chair to this chair. You know, you don't realise the thought it takes to think 'Now, how do I get him from point A to point B?'
Mr H: It's easy normally you just say 'I'll get out of bed and swing into there.' We have to spend half the afternoon thinking it out. If I didn't

have that hoist I'd never get from the bed to the wheelchair, you can't even get up. You see, if you've got hands you can do it you can lift yourself up and down with hands and arms but when you get like this it's very difficult.

Mrs R also spent all of her time in bed or in her wheelchair and disliked the latter because it was not very comfortable. She could not get onto the settee or into an armchair because the arrangement of the room meant that the hoist could not be put in the right position, and there were disadvantages in using the one chair which was appropriately placed and accessible.

Mrs R: If it's a special occasion and I want to sit in that chair I have to use the hoist to get in and out of it but I don't like doing that because once I'm in that chair I'm stuck you see and if there are people here you don't like bringing the hoist out and getting in it in front of people. That's my fault. It's vanity, I suppose, it isn't a nice feeling.

Mrs R disliked using the hoist even when there was no one there to watch. Three years prior to the interview the hoist had broken while in use, and she had fallen to the floor. More recently her daughter had noticed one of the links in the chain was pulling apart and fearing another accident had tried repeatedly without success to have someone come to effect a repair. For the past three months, the hoist had been used as little as possible, and Mrs R had reduced her number of baths from four to one a week: 'Naturally I was frightened and my bath day was agony 'cus I used to dread getting into that hoist but I knew I'd got to have that bath.' The day prior to the interview the hoist had broken again, but luckily Mrs R had been over the bed at the time and had not been hurt by the fall. She had also started to get what she described as 'panicky feelings' and attributed this in part to her absolute dependence upon mechanical aids.

Mrs R: I don't understand what they are . . . it's a trapped feeling because after being bedridden for years I did get walking but I was so much younger then and I didn't have the weight. I mean Saturday I had one and that was looking at the hoist, you know, and I thought, 'O God, I'm so reliant on that,' you know, and if my chair isn't next to me I get a little bit panicky over that. It is a little bit frightening.

Getting in and out of a chair was equally a problem for those who retained the ability to walk. Ordinary furniture was either too low or too soft so that the person sank to a position from which it was difficult to rise. Some had acquired special chairs through their rehabilitation officer, and Mrs V had spent £280 to buy herself an electrically operated chair recommended by a man she met while on holiday at a centre for disabled people. She had been given £300 by the local authority after being rehoused and decided to use it 'to get a bit of comfort for myself'. In public places the respondents would seek out hard chairs with high backs and would choose a kitchen stool or dining room chair in preference to an apparently more comfortable armchair. Down at the pub, Mr I always used a bar stool; they were so high he could slip on and off and never needed to ask for help.

Washing and bathing

All but three of the respondents needed help of one kind or another with washing and bathing, and of those one, Mrs N, had only recently begun to manage by herself. Bathing was so difficult that some would avoid it altogether or only bath when someone else was present, and all had aids to assist them to get into and out of the bath or to make it easier to wash once in. The nature of the problem varied from person to person; some could get into the bath but not out, some out but not in, and some had to be assisted both getting in and getting out. Nearly all found that certain areas of the body were inaccessible and either left them unwashed or were helped by spouses, daughters, or friends. Mrs W had one bath a week on a Saturday or Sunday when her husband was at home to operate the hoist. The other days she washed herself as best she could using a sponge on a long stick and only asked a friend to come round to do her back and hair if she were going out. For some, the problems varied from day to day according to where they had pain. Mrs A found that there was always some part of the body which could not be reached, and as this shifted from day to day, it was difficult to design a strategy to cope. Shaving was a particular problem for the men. Mr H was shaved by his wife, Mr I had a friend come to shave him because Mrs I could not manage the job, and Mr F could shave himself but only by virtue of a great deal of effort: 'I do eventually finish but it's hard work.' The women had to be helped with hair care and found commercial hairdressers inaccessible or otherwise difficult to use. Mrs A had often become so stiff sitting under the dryer that it was then very difficult for her to walk across the salon and even more difficult getting back home. Mrs G was more fortunate; her son was a hairdresser and would do her hair every time he called. Some, however, did without or relied on amateurs. Mrs R said 'This friend said "I'll make you look nice, I'll come and perm your hair." And, my God, she did. We couldn't get the comb through it and we still can't, but these are the things you have to put up with.'

Again, fairly elaborate strategies were developed in order to undertake tasks which ordinarily would require little planning or forethought. Mr F used a combination of aids and help to get in and out of the bath and also had a technique which meant he could manage on his own on a good day.

Mr F: I've got a seat I use in the bath so I make it a four stage, you know. Sit on the side, get my legs in, sit on the seat, then down into the bath, and somebody takes the seat out for me. I have a bath and do the opposite coming out. Then again if I feel all right I'm sometimes able to get up without the seat. I use my elbow on the edge of the bath and I get a towel or something, usually I use the rubber mats from my car 'cus they're rubber and they don't slip and I hang one of those over the side and I get my elbow on that and I can put most of my weight on my elbow and get up. It's a bit of a job but if I'm stuck waiting to get out of the bath that's the best way to do it.

Those who lived alone either made do with a wash down and took the opportunity of having a bath if they visited relatives or friends or had a district nurse or bathing attendant call once a week to assist them. Mr P only ever had a bath if he visited his sister-in-law and the rest of the time managed as best he could.

Int: Do you have trouble bathing?
Mr P: Dead trouble . . . I fear going in there. I'm afraid one day I'm going to get trapped in there, you know, what I do now is just stand in the bath. Luckily when I came here I changed the bath taps and put a shower on and that's all I do now.
Int: What's the difficulty?
Mr P: I can get in the bath but I have a job to get out. If I happen to sit on the edge of the bath if it's wet I try to remember to put a towel there to sit on. If it happens to be wet I go straight to the floor and get jammed between the bath and the floor and bang my head and all sorts.

Mrs V and Miss B lived alone and had to rely on formal help. This meant fitting in with the routine of the provider, but at least they got a bath.

Miss B: She don't come till one o'clock so I'm sitting in me dressing gown till then and I hate that, I like to get dressed straight away. Still, you can't have it all ways, they're so busy.

Getting dressed

For people with limited movement in their arms and shoulders, an inability to bend, and little in the way of manual dexterity, getting in and out of clothing may be impossible. The majority of the respondents found some aspect of dressing and undressing to be a problem even though clothes were purchased which had front zips and fastenings, were loose fitting and easy to climb into. The extent and nature of the problem varied from person to person. Mr S could manage to dress and undress and only had trouble with heavy winter coats. Mrs A had trouble with zips and buttons but got her husband to fasten her dress before he left for work. Mr

F found jackets his only problem. If he wanted to go out, he would carry his jacket downstairs, hoping to find someone in the flats below to give him a hand; when he got back his jacket would have to stay on until someone came home to help him get it off. Mr S could dress the upper part of his body but everything below the waist had to be dressed by his wife. He needed extensive help everyday. For some, dressing and undressing was a major problem, sometimes taking as long as an hour despite ingenious methods and improvised aids. Mrs V and Mrs W had the most difficulty.

Mrs V: Dressing? Oh don't. Dressing and undressing is a nightmare, believe me it is. I very seldom change once I'm dressed in the morning and wherever I'm going it's got to stop on because it's such an effort to dress. I have to stop in my stockings because I can't take them off and I can't put them on so they have to be on for a week at a time and the nurse changes them when she comes to bath me.

Int: What sort of problems do you have?

Mrs V: It's underclothes mostly. I have to use the handle of me stick to get me knickers on, yes it's a game. When I was on holiday I had to share the bedroom with another woman and she was in a wheelchair and yet to see her put her tights on in the morning. I used to say to her 'Gawd, I wish to God I could do that.' Well, one day, you don't like embarrassing yourself in front of other people, she went down to the toilet and while she's gone I thought to myself 'I'll put some clean knickers on' and while I was in the middle of putting them on she came back, so she got in the door and she stood there and she laughed and laughed her head off. She said 'I don't know, the tricks we people have to get up to.' She said 'I've never seen anything like it in my life.' I said 'Well, if you can't do it one way you've got to find another way of doing these things.'

Int: What were you doing?

Mrs V: Trying to pull my knickers up with me walking stick. That's the tragedy of trying to dress, it's shocking, no one would believe it.

Int: How long does it take you to get dressed in the morning?

Mrs W: Oh I get up around eight I suppose and I'm still trying to get dressed by nine. Sometimes I get so agitated because it's difficult to get dressed, my arms kill me, they really do, and I think 'Don't bother, don't bother yourself, why am I bothering? I'll sit here all day like some people do.' And then I think 'Somebody's coming,' and it sort of bucks me up. I can quite understand elderly people when they are like me sit in a chair and don't move 'cus you do feel like it, it's very painful. So it takes me all that time and all the time I'm looking at the clock thinking 'God!' So then if somebody rings me or interrupts my flow of getting ready it puts me all out again. I've got to stick to my routine.

Mrs T also managed to dress with the assistance of improvised aids. Because she could not bend, stockings were a problem but one which could be overcome. The stocking applicators she had tried all proved to be hopeless, and she had made her own out of two pieces of tape with suspender attachments sewn on the ends. These were clipped to the top of the stocking which was thrown on the floor, the foot inserted and the stocking pulled to the top of the leg.

Household management

The kinds of physical skills needed to successfully accomplish tasks like washing and dressing must be supplemented by others if the activities involved in managing a household are to be mastered. Ordinary activities such as cooking, cleaning, and shopping demand the ability to bend, kneel, reach, climb, lift and carry, push and pull, and the ability to manipulate delicate and heavy objects. The majority of people with rheumatoid arthritis have lost or are in the process of losing some, if not all of these skills. The loss of strength in limbs and joints means that apparently simple jobs like ironing and polishing cannot be completed and heavier work like hanging curtains or decorating must be abandoned altogether. It is not surprising then that all but one of the respondents were forced to accept help with their domestic duties.

Eight of the twenty-four respondents had a local authority home help and two more paid for their own. Of those living alone, six had a home help, two received help from family and friends, and one, Miss Z, had no help at all. The remainder attempted to do as much as they could but largely relied on spouses and/or daughters either living in the household or living elsewhere. The wives of the disabled men tended to provide all the assistance necessary while the husbands of disabled women were more likely to share the management of the household with daughters. While sons might help with heavy jobs, they were not conspicuous as providers of domestic help. The amount of help needed and received varied from respondent to respondent. Mrs J did nearly everything, including scrubbing floors and the laundry for a family of seven, while Miss L tidied and did a little dusting but nothing more. Mr P, who lived alone, had a home help for two hours a week while Mrs T's home help worked for six hours even though she had a husband who was also willing to help.

Few of the respondents were able to do much in the way of cleaning; like Miss L, tidying and dusting were about their limit. Attempts at polishing only produced a mess, and vacuum cleaners were generally too heavy to lift and push. Mrs A had bought a lightweight model in the hope of being able to continue to clean but found it to require more effort than an ordinary one. She had also been supplied with a lightweight iron and found that to be useless; it required such pressure to be effective that it was more difficult to wield than an ordinary one. Consequently, when she ironed clothes she did it only for short periods of time. This strategy of doing a little often was used by all of those who still retained responsibility for the housework. It was for this reason that Mrs J cleaned every day.

Mrs J: It's very seldom that I don't hoover the hall and this room every day. My husband says to me sometimes, 'Oh, leave it and do it tomorrow.' What people don't realize is that it's the same with me washing, if I leave it for two days that's a terrible lot to do and it's hard work but I do a little bit and then it's only a little bit I've got to do everyday then that's fine but if you leave it, if I leave this room for a couple of days it gets right grubby, to me it's hardly worth it to clear up three days in one than do it each day. It might not make sense to you but it does to me.

The only other alternatives are not to bother cleaning at all or to hand over the job to someone else. Miss Z lived alone, had no home help and few visitors and was able to be somewhat pragmatic about housework: 'I clean when I feel like it, you don't need to if you've no visitors, you only need to clean if people are coming.' Mrs A managed the problem by lowering her standards and reducing the need for housework.

Mrs A: I manage but it's probably not very efficient. There's a lot I can't do but I'm learning to turn my back on that a bit which I expect you find with other people. You've got to otherwise I think you'd go mad. As you can see looking around I'm afraid I've got an attitude do it now. Well, hard luck, if it doesn't get polished, it doesn't get polished.

Even when the task is taken over by someone else, standards may have to be lowered in order to bring them into line with the helper's way of going about things. Mrs N found this was necessary in order to avoid conflict in the family.

Mrs N: My husband doesn't like ironing, so it mounts up. I sometimes get angry but I can't say anything because it's not his job to be doing it and it's not my daughter's job to have to come in from work and see to me. It's frustration really, you see a pile of ironing and you just have to wait until one of them feels like doing it. At first I used to ask them to do it I got so frustrated but after a while you learn to curb it 'cus you've upsetting everybody else as well as yourself. I realized it wasn't fair on them so I've learnt to take it as it comes. I don't let it worry me now seeing jobs not done. Life's too short to be bothered with petty things like that.

While cleaning may be ignored and a degree of domestic disarray tolerated, shopping for food is an essential activity and cannot be avoided. Consequently, all had developed some arrangement for making sure they were supplied with essential goods. Those living alone had the most difficulty as did those without relatives or friends upon whom they could call. Because they rarely had access to private transport and because home helps could not be asked to travel to major shopping centres, they were forced to patronize the relatively expensive local shops and could not take advantage of cheaper prices elsewhere. Miss Z was able to get to the local shops and rested on walls on the way there and back in order to allow pain to subside. She managed by planning ahead; every time she went to the shop she bought a few additional items over and above her immediate needs and kept her cupboards well stocked. These reserves were used when the weather was bad, and she could not get out. She said 'You have to plan ahead if you live alone and there's no one you can depend on.' Mr P was unable to get to the shops and left all his shopping to the home help. Weekends were often a problem as he was unable to replace goods that ran out or fetch what had been forgotten. If he happened to see a neighbour passing the door he would ask him or her to collect whatever he needed; otherwise he would have to do without. Mrs Q occasionally went shopping with a friend but would never go alone: 'I wouldn't trust myself going round the shops, you could fall or the lifts can give out and then it's trouble for everybody.' A friend came twice a week to help with shopping, and on the days Mrs Q went to a luncheon club, the able-bodied there would buy her groceries which were carried home with her in the ambulance.

Shopping posed much less of a problem for those with spouses or daughters to help. Husbands would accompany wives and do all the lifting and carrying or go out on a Saturday morning and buy everything that was needed for the following week. Daughters would arrive with cars to take disabled parents to major shopping centres, and disabled men with cars would take their wives to the shops and collect them when the job was completed. Mrs J was unable to carry heavy shopping bags so would take a push chair to the nearest supermarket and load her provisions into that. Her husband or one of her daughters would meet her in order to push it back: 'I can push it on the flat but going up and down kerbs with a pram load of shopping I can't. I haven't got the strength in my wrists.' If no one was at home to help, she would buy a few items at the local shops where prices were high or would have to manage her main shopping alone.

Mrs J: Mostly my husband comes and meets me but if he has to go to the hospital or the doctor there are times I have to do it myself. Now walking down there with the push chair with nothing on it is marvellous, I'm dancing along as though I haven't got a care in the world, but you should see me coming back. Last week I went round the whole of Brixton and as I came back there's little side roads and I stood there and counted the ups and downs, there's four or five roads, and I thought there's no way I'm going to do that and I marched myself out into the gutter and walked up in the gutter facing the oncoming traffic till I got to the last of the ups and downs. They must have thought I'd gone crackers.

In this way Mrs J managed to get the shopping done despite the cost to her public identity.

Other household tasks like cooking or doing the laundry were also more complicated for those living alone. The difficulty of preparing a meal meant that they survived on a combination of meals on wheels, meals provided at centres or luncheon clubs, simple things they were able to prepare themselves, and food prepared by their home help. Mrs G was typical.

Mrs G: What I'm doing now is meals on wheels seven days a week. I drown most of them in Worcester sauce just to give them a little spunk, they come for everybody's taste and National Health teeth won't get through that meat. I make breakfast which simply consists of toast, coffee, and luncheon meat. A dietician's hair would probably stand on end but that's protein and roughage. In the evening I have convenience foods, it's an expensive way of doing things but I've very little option you see now I have the combination of no legs, no eyes, and no feeling, there's no question of cooking. I've trained my home help to leave me a salad big enough so it'll last for two days, so I've little more to do than go to the fridge and get it out. You see, by having to prepare food and do things one normally does oneself we're taking time that could be spent in cleaning and ironing, so it just doesn't happen.

Where cooking was possible it was limited to what could be achieved on the top of the stove and might be even more limited by an inability to lift and manipulate heavy objects. Mrs Q never boiled vegetables since she could not manage to strain them and avoided anything that could constitute a danger to herself. Ovens were not used by many for that very reason; having to bend to remove hot dishes from the oven was either impossible or just too risky. The diets of the respondents tended to be monotonous and lack variety unless there was someone there to help. Mrs A did what she could in the kitchen but was forced to leave many tasks to her husband: 'I don't know what I'd do if I hadn't got him around. To be quite honest I'd probably have to live on something very simple.' Ingenuity sometimes triumphed over physical difficulty and allowed an individual to find ways around the problem of preparing favourite foods. Mrs W could not reach the eye level grill from her wheelchair but could reach the oven. She was addicted to cheese on toast and found that by using an electric toaster, melting the cheese in the oven and assembling the components at a later stage, she could produce a version which met her previous standards.

The cost of doing laundry or the need to depend on others was often reduced by doing some at home and only sending heavy articles elsewhere to be washed. Mrs Q washed light articles everyday so that it did not pile up, and the rest was taken by a friend to a local launderette. Where laundry was not sent away or done by others and where no machine was available at home, there was often no option other than to do the lot by hand. Mr P found launderettes expensive and could not rely on there being anyone available to give him a hand. Consequently, he left his washing to soak in the bath and managed as best he could. Sheets and towels were a big problem as this method was both laborious and inefficient. But without the necessary resources at hand, he just had to put up with a job that was not well done.

While all of the respondents had little choice but to depend upon others, not all were happy at having to ask for help. The married women in particular disliked having to hand over domestic duties to husbands and daughters. They saw managing the household as their job and an inability to perform in this respect was one of the ways chronic illness caused them to fail in a valued role. This was the case even when housework did not appear to be resented by spouses and offspring. It was because of this sense of role that Mrs J struggled to retain her control over domestic affairs, and Mrs W chose to pay herself for domestic help. Mrs W thought it unfair to expect her husband to come home from work to have to clean the house, and Mrs J, while willing to accept help, was not prepared to be dependent upon others.

> *Mrs J:* My kids have to come home from work and do ironing every night and my little one, she's fourteen, she has to take her turn of ironing and Saturday they all help me clean this house. Now that's fair enough, I believe in families helping. I believe in kids doing their share, but what I don't believe in is my having to put a greater burden on them, such as they do a day's work they don't want to come home to housework, not if their mother's at home all the time and I've always been at home.

The apparently mundane tasks involved in managing a household are of significance and value to those women who have adopted the role of wife and mother and see their life's work as caring for others. Chronic illness and physical disability turn this situation upside down, make them recipients rather than the providers of care and leaves them with a deep sense of loss. Mrs R, now totally dependent upon her daughter, said 'I loved it when I could do my housework, it was painful but I loved it all the same. Now I can't do it it's pretty awful. A mother has a child to take care of not the other way round.' Similarly, Mrs J's main worry was how long she was going to be able to maintain her role: 'How long I'm going to be able to keep going and keep my home clean, whether I'll be able to get up in the morning and do my housework to the way I want it that's what worries me.'

Mobility

Seven of the respondents were sufficiently mobile to be able to walk about outside the house without the help of others, although three of these could only walk for short distances before they were forced to rest to allow pain to subside. One other, Mrs K, could walk about outside if she was accompanied and supported by her husband. The remainder could not or did not walk around outside at all. Some of these were capable of walking for short distances but would not go out unless they were able to use a car. Four of the people needed a wheelchair out of doors. Twelve of the respondents had easy access to a car; they either owned one, one was owned by a spouse or child living in the household or one was owned by a close relative not in the household who could be called upon at any time. At times *all* respondents experienced some difficulty in moving about inside their flat or house, let alone outside.

Apart from the four confined to wheelchairs, two other respondents always needed some form of aid to help them get around inside, though at times would make use of a stick. Mr S and Miss B used walking frames, and both found some difficulty in manoeuvring in small places like the bathroom and toilet. Miss B preferred to use a small tea trolley to assist her to get around and found it doubly useful in that it carried all the paraphernalia she might need during the day. Some of the respondents found sticks difficult to use, causing discomfort in the hand or shoulder, and on bad days were forced to spend most of their time in a chair. Mr I was hoping for a wheelchair to improve his mobility indoors, but Mrs G used hers with the greatest reluctance: 'The whole flat is about 20 feet square and that's about all I can manage. I've got a wheelchair. Hurray! I'm not going in a wheelchair. I'm not staying in one. No way.' Weak arms and hands made it difficult for some to get around even in a wheelchair so that Mrs T had to propel herself along with her feet. She had recently been supplied with an electric chair, the latest flare-up having resulted in an inability to use one leg. She was not finding it easy to control and after falling out of it several times thought she might send it back. Mr H had use of neither arms nor legs and had to be pushed around even indoors. When his wife took him down to the nursing unit, he often found himself placed in the television room: 'It's extremely hot with the heating on and all I can do is sit there and gasp. If the nurses are busy or having their tea then I'm stuck.' His doctor was arranging for him to be supplied with an electric chair so that he could move about indoors unaided and perhaps make use of the grounds around his flat.

Stairs and steps inside the house were, of course, a major problem. Four people lived in houses and had to use an internal staircase, three lived above the second floor in buildings with no lifts and three in buildings with lifts. The rest were fortunate in that by accident or design they lived in ground floor flats. Steps and stairs required a special technique if they were to be negotiated successfully. Mrs X always came down stairs backwards, and Mrs J would come down in a similar manner if she was in pain and wished to avoid any stress on her knees and feet. Most of the time she would manage by coming down sideways, sliding down the supporting wall. Going up stairs was less of a problem since arms as well as legs could be employed. Mrs A and Mr M both lived in flats which could only be reached by climbing fifty-two steps. Mr M was accommodated in a large complex of local authority housing and, by planning his route and walking around the entire block to the lifts, he could avoid thirty of those steps. Not so for Mrs A who had to climb down and back up the entire fifty-two every time she went out.

> *Mrs A:* The thing is you get a technique. Even when I'm bad I never have both legs bad at the same time not, you know, really stiff so I can't move either and I find that by dint of putting one down first and then the other I can manage. The way I go down stairs it's like a child you know, one step at a time.

Despite having developed a technique for getting down stairs, it did involve quite a considerable loss of time. Some days it took her ten minutes to get from the door of the flat down to street level. Consequently, she only ever went out for a good reason and usually only once a day.

Some of those able to walk about outside would often not bother because of the pain it caused and the need for frequent rests which made progress unacceptably slow. Mr F rarely went out unless he was able to use his car.

> *Mr F:* You see, literally as soon as I stand up my knee gets me and down this ankle, but to walk about 400 feet then I've got to sit down, you know, I've got to do something or stand up and hang on, you know, just to take the weight off my feet. After a few minutes I can start off again and plod off again and do that on and off, on an' off. So it takes me about twenty minutes to walk about 200 yards.

Mrs X was able to walk to and from the local luncheon club but rarely attempted to go further afield: 'If I walk any distance for about fifteen minutes I'm really done up. It's sheer misery and it's not worth it.' Once again, pain could be avoided or minimized but only at a price, in this case being independently mobile only within the confines of a limited geographical boundary.

Mobility around the community is made more difficult and often limited by the structure of the physical environment. This is so, irrespective of whether or not the person must use a wheelchair. Even those who retained the ability to walk outside the home encountered a number of obstacles during their journeys around the area in which they lived. The most significant obstacle was kerbs, largely because they are so numerous that any walk seemed to involve negotiating one or two, and their frequency made them difficult if not impossible to avoid altogether. The step down from the pavement to the road, although only a matter of inches, had to be managed very carefully and demanded the same kind of techniques used to cope with steps and stairs; the person must stop at the edge of the kerb and go down one foot at a time. This was particularly difficult in a busy street because it conflicted with the continuous flow of pedestrian traffic. Some had been knocked over since such changes in flow had not been anticipated by the hurrying non-disabled. One or two found kerbs impossible to manage, and Mr S, on the rare occasions he walked outside, needed to be helped down and pushed up by his wife. The problem could sometimes be minimized by planning and routing (Fagerhaugh 1973), identifying, and using particular pathways through the community.

> *Mr M:* I always plan the way I go so there's very little kerbs or anything like that. If I go along the Brixton Road where the crossings are it's not so bad, there it's all smooth so I have to plan. I go up that way to try and avoid it.

As basic strategies, planning and routing not only reduce the physical difficulty of moving around the community, they also do so in a manner which helps to preserve the person's public identity. By avoiding obstacles they can only negotiate awkwardly or in the manner of an incompetent such as a child, persons with arthritis can more easily conceal their illness and disability. Techniques which are used for moving around in the privacy of the home may be unacceptable in public places since they constitute a threat to identity. It has often been reported that many people with mobility problems refuse to use aids such as walking sticks or wheelchairs because it labels them disabled, and this was equally true of some of the respondents here. Mrs G's refusal to accept a wheelchair was not derived from a desire to appear normal in public; she had been blind for a number of years and willingly carried a white stick. Rather, it stemmed from her refusal to give in and accept that she would no longer be independently mobile. The meaning of such aids was quite different for Mrs A who had been advised to use a walking stick.

> *Mrs A:* I would rather not . . . it's part vanity but also I've normally a handbag and a small shopping bag and I think I would find a stick an

added encumbrance. So, no . . . not really. You do feel, you know, and I expect other people have told you this, if you have any disability of this kind you do feel very second class and I think most people are very very anxious to appear as normal as possible. I think giving in to a walking stick would be one very retrograde step and I'd rather not at the moment. When I have to I will.

Not all respondents took this point of view. Others, like Mrs W, were prepared to trade a good public identity for increased mobility. This may have been because she was already confined to a wheelchair and had no good identity to lose. She was sufficiently mobile within her flat but once out of doors could go no further than the point where the path from her front door met the pavement. She had seen people using a Batricar, an elaborate electric wheelchair powerful enough to master pavements and slopes.

> *Mrs W:* I'd like one of those things so I could go along the pavement, 'cus I would use it, I don't worry about people looking at me, I'd just go out in it but unfortunately I've never been offered one.

Those confined to wheelchairs found the physical environment even more problematic and could not manage without having someone to push. In spite of such help, there were still severe limits on how far they could go. A simple trip to the local High Street created a number of difficulties for Mr H and his wife.

> *Mr H:* The fumes are shocking, the petrol and diesel fumes along the High Road. I can hardly get a hundred yards in the fumes and I'm gasping for breath so she has to take me all round the back streets. There's so many slopes and hills that that's a battle to get up and down, either the wheelchair's running away or she's puffing and panting to push it back up the hill. We find this very frustrating all this carry on. It's too much of a struggle for her so we're restricted to what route we go and how far we go.

A further limitation was imposed because of Mr H's need to use the toilet. This was such a problem that he had asked at the hospital if there was any kind of aid to help. He had seen a woman wearing a catheter and urine bag and thought something of that kind would be ideal for him.

> *Mr H:* I asked 'Do you supply any gadget I can use when I want to go to the toilet 'cus if I'm out on the High Road in the Gents toilet and there's nobody there so the wife's got to push me into the Gents and I can't use the damn toilet in any case?' I said 'Is there not some kind of internal plastic bag or something if I want to use the other end?' and he said 'No.' You see, simple things become a nightmare. In the hospital we've found a little toilet in the Rheumatology Department she can take me

into, she can't take me into the Gents. Then we can manage you see, she can give me a bottle. But you can't do that on Streatham High Road. You can't do that in the Gents. So I've got to say 'Quick. You've got half an hour's rush to get me home.'

Because of these difficulties some of the respondents simply stayed at home; they went out only if they were collected by car or ambulance and returned home at the end of the trip. This, of course, required access to resources such as persons willing to help, private transport, or the facilities provided by welfare agencies.

Only a minority of the respondents used public transport and then only when it was absolutely necessary. They would use buses during off-peak hours when they were not so crowded or wait for an empty bus to come along so they could be sure of getting a seat. One difficulty shared by all was getting on and off the bus, though this might be better or worse according to the tolerance of bus conductors and officials. When Mrs G used to travel by bus to work for the Blind Society, she always found conductors helpful and willing to assist. Mr C, who had no official badge such as a white stick, was not so lucky and had encountered many people who were not prepared to bend the rules to make life easier for him.

Mr C: Some of them'll let you stand on the platform at the back of the bus but more of them'll tell you to get off you can't stand there. I could sit down if I could get on but there's another step up there you know, there's one as you get on then another, you've got to hold on to that bar, they won't give you time you see, they move off straight away.

Mrs Q also found that public transport presented a number of insurmountable barriers and was out of the question.

Mrs Q: I can't get on and off buses and even if I could the bus stop is so far away I would have to take the wheelchair and I know no buses will take me with the chair on. But even if I could get on the buses I'd still have to have somebody with me to help me, and there is no one.

It was very frustrating to Mrs Q that she was 'unable to go from A to B on me own' without having to spend scarce financial resources on a taxi. She had a friend with a car who was willing to take her wherever she wanted to go but it was still necessary to wait until it was convenient for him. She had reached an age where she was eligible for a free bus pass but was unable to take advantage of the concession because of the problems involved. She did not receive a mobility allowance or any other compensatory payment; compared to her peers she was doubly disadvantaged.

Housing and the immediate physical environment
Some of the data in the previous section illustrates the point that disability

and disadvantage are very much influenced by the physical environment in which chronically sick persons live. This environment has for the most part been constructed with little or no sensitivity to the needs of people who are impaired in some way and often means they cannot use the skills they retain or have developed in order to pursue valued activities (Shearer 1981). The immediate context is handicapping where it presents barriers which must be negotiated, consuming reserves of time, money, and energy in the process, or where the effort is such the person decides not to bother and retreats into an enforced passivity. It is also handicapping to the extent it leaves the individual with no option but to rely on the help of others. Housing is, of course, a very important part of the physical environment since its character and layout may promote or impede the person's ability to perform the essential, though mundane, activities of everyday life as and when he or she wishes. It is, perhaps, the easiest part of the environment to modify in accordance with individual needs.

Twelve of the twenty-four people interviewed were living in housing they had been allocated or had acquired by virtue of their disability. This had been specially built or partially adapted for the disabled or elderly or consisted of a conventional flat located at ground floor level. Prior to the move some had lived in their own homes and had given them up because they were too large or otherwise unmanageable, and some had lived in rented accommodation which was unsuitable for a variety of reasons. Three had ground floor flats which had been occupied prior to their becoming disabled, two continued to live in their own house or the house of a relative, and seven lived in accommodation which was unsuitable, either because it was in very poor condition, was not adapted in any way, or was in a block without lifts. Of these seven, four were waiting to be rehoused, and three were considering applying to the local authority for better accommodation. The ones living in the worst circumstances tended to be those who occupied houses or flats owned by the local authority or Greater London Council in streets or complexes which were gradually being emptied prior to demolition or renovation. Their living space was small, lacked basic amenities, and was badly affected by damp. Moreover, no adaptations had been undertaken owing to their 'impending move', and they were situated in areas with a lot of derelict and boarded property, giving the area a neglected and depressing air.

Not all of those who had recently moved, or were wanting to move, lived in accommodation in a poor state of repair. Mrs W and Mrs A had previously lived in privately rented flats which they liked, and Mr M currently occupied a new local authority flat with a large balcony. In each case the problem had been stairs. Mrs W had occupied a flat on the first floor of a large Victorian house with the added disadvantage of three steps in the middle of the corridor joining the lounge and kitchen to the bedroom and bathroom. Once confined to a wheelchair she was carried into the kitchen every morning and spent most of the day there. Because the bathroom was inaccessible, it had been necessary for her to use a commode placed on the landing. The advantage of the flat was the kitchen; totally rebuilt by her husband, all the cupboards and surfaces were within easy reach. The specially adapted flat in which she now lived had a conventional kitchen which was impossible for her to use. At the first interview, Mrs A was still living in a flat which could only be reached by a climb of fifty-two steps and managed by carefully planning her day so as to make constant journeys up and down unnecessary. Even that was proving too much and by the time of the second interview the A's had moved to a flat on the ground floor which had many advantages but some disadvantages.

Mrs A: I can't drive as much as I did but I do go out rather more. And also if I happen to forget something at the shops I don't sit and think 'Oh blow, we'll go without', I can go and get it. It's a great advantage in that respect. I'm sure it's better for me not having to climb stairs. I don't like the surroundings very much. I know this sounds awfully snobby but I never imagined I'd end up on a council estate, but I mean, what choice does one have? Beggars and arthritics can't be choosers. I couldn't have gone on, I know, at the other flat, I would like to have as I liked the flat very much but it was just impossible it had to be a move otherwise I would have been sitting in all day and that was that.

At the first interview, Mr M was managing despite a similar climb up fifty-two steps to his flat; there was a lift he could use part of the way at the end of a short walk. By the time of the second interview the lift had been vandalized so often it had been sealed up and was no longer in use.

Mr M: I've got to face the fact of being stuck in here eventually or get a ground floor flat where you can just pop out 'cus the effort of getting down the steps is a bit dodgy 'cus the old hands are going. I've spent a lot of money on this flat, there was £1000 for that carpet and I won't get the benefit of that. Half of this stuff won't probably fit in and there's no way I can replace it. It'd break my heart to leave 'cus there's a lot of work gone into this place.

The specially built or adapted housing units in which some of the respondents were currently living had many advantages, the main one being that the flats were on the ground floor and on one level. Though this promoted mobility around the home, it was not to everyone's liking. Mrs X had requested and been allocated a small house; she preferred the struggle of climbing stairs to the insecurity of having to sleep on the ground floor. Mrs I had asked to be moved from their damp ground floor flat to a house. Her plan was to accommodate her disabled husband on the ground floor and her children in the upstairs rooms where they would disturb him less. There were some advantages to be gained from the specific changes made in order to better accommodate a disabled person. Bath rails, high toilets, doors wide enough to take a wheelchair, doors that opened both ways and did not have to be pulled, and switches and sockets placed at a convenient height all made a difference to daily living. Some of the benefits were incidental and not a product of adaptations or special design. Mrs A liked having access to her own garden; she never went on holiday because of the cost and the difficulty of coping in the strange environment of a hotel and found using the garden during good weather an acceptable substitute. Mrs X and Mrs V now had access to a bathroom and hot running water, and Mrs K, who used to share a large house with her daughter, son-in-law, and two grandchildren, found her existence to be far more peaceful after she had moved. It is a pity then that many of these advantages were outweighed by the problems these special environments posed.

Some of the disadvantages the respondents encountered following their move to adapted housing stemmed from basic faults in design, and some arose because the housing had been adapted for disabled people in general and not individuals with particular needs. Some of the problems could be solved with a little work and some with the help of additional aids. Many, however, could not, and these were very much resented by the people who had no choice but to live with them, especially if they could and should have been avoided. For example, the back door to Mrs R's flat had been placed so as to make it very difficult for a wheelchair to pass through, and the garden could only be reached by going down two steps. Consequently, she had to be helped out into the garden and helped when she wanted to come back in again. In addition, while electric points had been installed to enable a hoist to be used, the ceilings in the bathroom and bedroom were not strong enough to take the weight of the mechanism. Mrs R made do with a portable hoist. Mrs A was unable to reach the windows in her flat and had to ask her husband to open or close them before he went to work, so they stayed as they were for the rest of the day. The changes to the bathroom were also of little help:

> *Mrs A:* Well they had this pole which I suppose theoretically was supposed to help you get off the loo or get into the bath. Well, for someone like me it was a dead loss I found that all it did I kept getting bruised by bumping into it and I found sitting on the loo it made it cramped so we've disposed of that. It has a low bath which is not much of a help because I already managed with my aids and it's much shorter than the other one which is a problem.

Her main complaint, however, was that in order to meet local fire regulations the doors in the flat had weighted chains attached to make them self closing.

Mrs A: Well, you can imagine what that did. Every time I pushed the kitchen door open it shut behind me and everytime I tried to come out with a tray I either threw the coffee on the floor or trapped my fingers. My husband went round with a screw driver and we've removed most of them. Then the council came round for their final inspection and said the borough surveyor would insist on them being put back so I said 'Well, if he does I shall take them off again and I shall go on with this until he gets really terse and takes me to court because I think it's nonsense.' They say it's a fire hazard but it's easier for me to get out and close the door behind me than to try and get out of the kitchen supposing I was stupid enough to burn a pan of fat or something I could be trapped in there quite easily with the chain on and not be able to open the door sufficiently because I've only got the power of a six-year old in one hand and I felt this was just stupid, it's more dangerous as it was.

One complaint mentioned by several women was that their flats seemed to have been designed for disabled men with able-bodied wives. The cupboards in Mrs R's kitchen had not been changed at all. All she could manage from her wheelchair was to put in plugs and switch on the light. When Mrs W moved from her upstairs flat with a kitchen to suit her needs to a ground floor flat with a conventional kitchen, she lost as much as she gained:

Mrs W: If the kitchen was like my other one I'd be fine because I could have my working top around me with my things on, there would be more space to turn the chair and I would have my sink which was low. My husband did all that for me. But now I can't . . . also the cupboards and everything's up high, I couldn't get anything out of them so really I couldn't really do anything for myself. It's all right probably if the husband's disabled with the wife doing the things but not with me trying to do what I'm doing. So actually, in a sense, it's done me no favours, it's took me away from doing the things I used to do.
Int: You miss that?
Mrs W: Yes, 'cus it gives you a sense of purpose that you've done something, you've gone round your kitchen, opened the cupboard, you've took the pan out. Now everything is done and put there which is not so good and I don't like it.

Even taking into account the problems still encountered by the people living in special or adapted housing, there is no doubt that they were much better off than all of those who did not. Many of those in conventional housing simply had to struggle on; moving from room to room to avoid damp which seemed to follow them around, coping with places too large to keep clean or too small for their needs, with inadequate toileting and bathing facilities and plugs and switches placed so that they could not be reached, and coping with ill-fitting doors which could not be opened once closed and gas fires with pilot lights that went out frequently and could not be relit until someone was found to help. Surprisingly, one or two were not so unhappy with these conditions that they had thought of being rehoused, and Mr P, though he disliked his small, dark flat and hated the dreary Victorian estate on which it was situated had not applied for special housing, believing that 'once you've got a place the council won't look at you'. Those waiting to be moved could not be more anxious to leave their current accommodation and hoped that a disabled person's flat would transform their everyday life. Their main concern was the area to which they would be moved; most wanting to stay near family and friends, highly regarded general practitioners, and local facilities such as shops. Mrs J, born and raised within the sound of the hooters from the barges on the Thames, in streets dominated by a railway viaduct and the noise from two iron foundries, would not contemplate a move up the hill to middle-class Streatham.

> *Mrs J:* I'll tell you why I don't like Streatham, why I wouldn't live up there, it's too big, I don't like great big places, but also, I don't know if you know Streatham. No? Well, you're not missing anything. You go up Brixton Hill into Streatham Hill and all the way along the roads off where people live, I think they must number up to 300, they're really long roads plus the fact they're all up hill and down dale. Now the council will think nothing of sticking me at the end of one of those roads. Now the shops are all down in Streatham Hill so it's pouring with rain, the kids are at work, there's only me, I've no shopping, I might get down the road to get the shopping but Christ knows how I get it back. It's bad enough here walking to Brixton and back. The thing is I'm not lazy, far from it but I'm used to home comforts. By home comforts I mean walk out of the top of this road I can get a bus anywhere. I like things on my doorstep so don't stick me up bleeding Streatham. You know, in that respect I'm selfish or spoilt, call it what you like. I walk across the flats up there and there's me doctor's so that suits me fine. You see that's another reason I don't want to move, I've got a marvellous doctor but I can't see him chasing up to the wilds of Streatham. Perhaps you could say I'm selfish in that my husband would love to live up there, but I bloody well ain't. I don't like quiet funnily enough. I'm happy to live on a main road. Well, I was born at Vauxhall, lived there all me life. In the street I lived had the railway one end, you always knew the time day and night and five doors away was an iron factory and a foundry at the other end of the street and my beautiful Thames. I still get a kick out of them boats as old as I am. I still love my Thames and my boats, you could hear all the sirens honking

on the water if it was foggy for one another to get out of the way. I was born to it and lived with it all my life. I don't like quiet, drives me crackers, so I'm not going to Streatham, I wouldn't live in Streatham rent free.

Whether Mrs J would have much of a choice was entirely another matter. Under the local housing regulations, prospective tenants were made three offers and then forced to accept the fourth, no matter how unsuitable or inconvenient.

The meaning of mundane activity

Few of us find much frustration in an inability to jump more than twenty feet, run a mile in under three and a half minutes, or successfully hit a heavily sliced cross court backhand. For most, the fact that such activities are beyond our capabilities is of little significance practically or symbolically; it has little impact on life in general and identity in particular. In this respect, mundane activities are significant simply because they are mundane; being unable to successfully bring off these tasks makes life extraordinarily difficult and has an impact on identity and self concept. It is a constant reminder that the individual is less than he or she once was. As Mrs N said, 'It's so frustrating when you can't do the things you used to sail through.' Similarly, at times, all of us encounter inanimate objects which seem to have a life of their own, refusing to bend to our will, or all of us occasionally have to be particularly careful with regard to the environment (Shearer 1981). When such experiences are sporadic, they are unlikely to have much of an influence on how we see ourselves; when they happen many times during the course of a day, it may be all too easy to see the problem as residing in our own incapacity rather than in objects or environments which have been constructed on the basis of unwarranted assumptions about peoples' needs. As Mr H said, 'I get annoyed. I get annoyed with myself, you know, that this sort of spirit is trapped within this useless body. I think, you know, "There must be an odd body kicking around that I can jump into." '

Some non-disabled, especially where they have sufficient financial resources, happily give over tasks such as shopping, cleaning, doing the laundry, and looking after the children to others. This transfer of essential but time-consuming and not particularly rewarding activities is a symbol of wealth if not power. The transfer of mundane tasks to others carries a different meaning for some disabled people; it is indicative of their incompetence to care for themselves or manage a household or move freely from A to B in the community, when others can take this for granted and easily accomplish the tasks they cannot do. Why else would Mrs J say 'I hate asking people to do things for me. I don't *want* other people to do things, I want to do them myself.'

Having to ask others to do things can involve several kinds of loss. This may vary from a loss of control over the activity, someone else decides how well and how often to do the cleaning, to a financial loss, as when Mr H said, 'Everything you want doing you have to pay somebody to do.' Being forced to have help with self care may be embarrassing or demeaning, as Mrs N discovered when she had to be bathed by her daughter, and Mrs R found when she had to be cleaned by her daughter after using the toilet. It may give rise to feelings of helplessness or dependency (see Chapter 6) or the feeling that your power to act upon and create within the world is being progressively lost. If you can't wash or dress yourself, what can you do? As Mrs D said, 'When you've been able to do all these things it hits you sometimes when you find you can't.' In a sense, the practical problems of everyday living are never solved; they are merely transformed. A relative may be happy and willing to do the shopping and cooking for a disabled person with the result that the recipient remains well fed but with a sense of guilt or feelings of being a burden, or it may cease being his or her problem and become one for someone else who has to reorganize his or her time to provide necessary assistance. Even where money is available to pay someone to do this sort of thing, it can still be annoying because, unlike the non-disabled, the disabled have no choice. It is perhaps for this reason that disabled people themselves put such emphasis on facilities and services designed to promote independent living (Shearer 1981). If the mundane practical problems of everyday life can be managed efficiently, time, energy, and money can be turned to the task of constructing a more satisfying existence based on access to social and other opportunities.

5 Work and income

For many disabled people becoming unemployed is a major transition point in their career. It not only marks the end of what may have been a painful and protracted struggle to remain in paid work, it radically transforms the character and pattern of their everyday lives and brings with it a host of other problems such as boredom, loss of social contracts, and loss of financial independence. Some of these problems are never wholly solved; however, over time, many diminish in significance as expectations and aspirations adjust or acquiesce to new realities. Consequently, it is among the recently unemployed where the lack of work and its social and material consequences are felt most acutely.

Of the respondents in this study all had worked at some time in their lives and all but two had given up work because of rheumatoid arthritis and its associated disability. Of these, eight people had been unemployed for three years or less, the remainder had been without paid work for between five and twenty years. Two of the men who were interviewed had occupied managerial positions, two had skilled manual jobs, and four had been unskilled workers such as lorry drivers. Of the women, one had been a nurse and more recently a teacher of the blind, three had held senior clerical positions, and the rest had done routine clerical work or had unskilled service occupations. At the time of the first interview only one, Miss L, was currently working although Mrs A was on extended sick leave from her job as a senior personal secretary in the Civil Service, and Mrs T operated a telephone answering service for a former employer who frequently travelled abroad. By the time of the second interview Mrs A had been retired by her employer and was thinking of looking for part-time work locally, and Mrs T had become almost bed-bound following an acute flare-up but still occasionally acted as messenger and receiver of telephone calls.

For the eight people who had been unemployed for three years or less, the lack of a job was regarded as a temporary state of affairs in the sense that they all expressed a desire to return to work. All, however, regarded their re-entry into the labour force as uncertain, either because it required a spontaneous or medically induced improvement in their condition or because it would be necessary to find a job and an employer sufficiently flexible to accommodate the erratic course of their condition and its effects. Some were at a critical stage in their lives in that the uncertainty surrounding their return to work needed to be resolved in order that they might have a clearer idea of their future prospects generally. Those who had been without jobs for longer periods of time seemed more often to view their situation as inevitable and had given up any thought of returning to paid work. They tended to see themselves as not working rather than unemployed, the older ones referring to themselves as retired. For these people, the problem was no longer one of trying to return to work but of finding acceptable alternative activities in order to keep occupied.

In Blaxter's (1976) study of 194 people disabled by a wide variety of conditions, two types of occupational career pattern were observed, those of discontinuity and drift. The former involved a sudden change from employed to unemployed and a rapid transformation in daily living, the latter a slow drift down the occupational scale through a series of jobs, each less satisfying and less well rewarded than the previous one until the final drift into unemployment. The dominant pattern among the people interviewed in this study was that of discontinuity; few evidenced downward drift over a prolonged period of time. Some, like Mr I and Mr M, became unemployed within months of onset while others, like Mrs A and Mr H, carried on working for 11 and 16 years respectively until their arthritis began to interfere both with daily life and work. During this time both had been promoted and both managed to carry on at work until forced to leave by sudden increases in pain and disability. One clear exception to this general pattern was Mr P. He was a skilled machine tool engineer prior to a sudden and very disabling onset and worked for a local engineering firm. On coming out of hospital he was unable to stand for long periods at the lathe or other machines and was given a job as an inspector checking the work of other men. When the firm went bankrupt he got a job in the local polytechnic setting up lathes and assisting students. He was asked to leave this job because of his disability and after one year's unemployment became a lift attendant. Although not an entirely suitable job for someone with rheumatoid arthritis, he stayed for 11 years and only left when all the lifts at work were made automatic. He was then advised to retire and gave up work at the age of 58.

As far as disabled persons are concerned, their occupational careers are likely to be structured by a number of factors, including the nature of the illness and the strategies required to manage it, the velocity of the illness trajectory, the nature of the work and the possibility that it can be reorganized in the face of disability, and the tolerance of workmates and employers. It is not unreasonable to suggest that the work histories of people with rheumatoid arthritis are likely to be characterized by discontinuity rather than drift since the illness is in many ways incompatible with the organization of work. Further, the character of the symptoms produced by the disease are likely to make it difficult to perform most if not all jobs, thereby minimizing the possibility of drift through a sequence of occupations. The main symptoms and consequences of rheumatoid arthritis which make it difficult to remain in the workforce are constant pain and loss of energy, limited mobility and manual dexterity, an inability to sit or stand for long periods without pain, and the fluctuating course of the illness requiring frequent absences from work. These combine to produce an erratic performance in the work role. Special working conditions or special relations with others at work are necessary to minimize these difficulties and their effects.

Problematic aspects of work

Quite obviously, the kinds of problems chronically sick and disabled people encounter at work depend upon the nature of the disorder from which they suffer, the nature of the task they are called upon to do and the nature of the physical and social environment in which they work. Some of these problems are related to the specific work task itself; others are identical to the more general practical problems of daily living. The extent to which these problems can be managed or solved determines whether or not the person concerned is able to remain at work. This may demand that the job be restructured to suit a person with reduced capabilities, that the environment be modified to remove physical barriers to effective performance, or it may require the assistance and co-operation of colleagues and those in authority. Consequently, whether or not the person continues to work is not a direct function of his or her location within the occupational hierarchy. Judging by the experience of those interviewed in this study, some managers and some manual labourers become unemployed soon after onset while some managers and some manual labourers are able to work for considerable lengths of time.

For the person suffering from rheumatoid arthritis, it is not necessarily the case that a so-called sedentary or clerical job is any less problematic than one which seemingly involves more physical labour. Limited mobility, an inability to lift and carry, the inability to sit for long periods of time, and the inability to accomplish tasks quickly disadvantage those who work in an office as much as those who are employed on the factory floor. For example, Mrs A was a secretary and found many aspects of her working life difficult.

Mrs A: The first problem I encountered was opening the swing doors into the department. Two sets push which are fine, you can use your whole body and that's not too difficult but two sets pull towards one and that I find very difficult. I used to find some of the staff there extremely unhelpful . . . they'd watch me put my shopping bag down and put my handbag down and grab the door with both hands and just tug and watch with interest. Erm . . . there are one or two rooms which can only be reached by stairs. I found that getting up and down stairs was difficult, lifts are fine. I found filing cabinets, pulling them open, very difficult. Audio plugs are frequently situated on the skirting under the central heating which I found very difficult, but I did just a few months before I went on sick leave manage to get two put on the wall which made life a lot easier. If I sat for any length of time I got terribly stiff and had to get up and walk around. I had an electric typewriter, I can't manage a manual one now. Reference books were difficult, you know. You would normally go to a book shelf and reach a book down. This is something I can't do. I have to very carefully take it down with two hands and quickly find somewhere to rest it. What else er . . . long treks round the building for photocopying and things like this. Again, there were sets of swing doors that needed to be pulled towards me, erm, perhaps pulling them an inch and a half and getting a foot in was a very cumbersome business. Occasionally I used to wait for somebody coming through them so that was OK.

Of course, those in manual occupations found their jobs problematic and recalled difficulties similar to those who did or had done non-manual work. This was the case even where the work was specifically intended for the disabled. Mr P worked for eleven years as a lift attendant:

Mr P: I took a job in the House of Commons operating the lifts but it nearly killed me sitting in the one position nearly 16 hours a day. When you came to move, when somebody came to relieve you, you couldn't move. You couldn't get out of the lift. In fact, I used to sit in the lift and go without my dinner rather than go through the pain of walking to dinner.

The extent to which doing a job is difficult depends in part on the specific circumstances under which it is performed. The same job in the same organization may prove easily manageable or impossible to do according to the demands of immediate superiors, the structure of the work situation, and the resources placed deliberately or fortuitously at the disabled person's disposal. Prior to her taking sick leave, Mrs A worked for a number of people.

Mrs A: I had an ideal situation until my boss retired actually, I had a room of my own. I had an electric typewriter, that was a great help. I had a messenger who was a motherly soul and if there were committee teas or anything always insisted on doing them and carrying them in 'cus I can't carry trays. I had at least three friends on the same corridor and if photocopying or anything was needed and they were on their way they quite often used to look in and say can they take it. . . ? It was a marvellous job situation but they don't happen very often.

When her boss retired Mrs A was allocated to someone else.

Mrs A: The situation was not as easy at all, in fact I finally had to ask for a transfer. I was working for a very busy and ambitious man and every Friday night regularly there were always submissions to the Minister that had to be carried round the department by hand and that meant going up and down stairs, in and out of lifts, and along corridors and finally I had to say 'I'm terribly sorry much as I like this job I can't keep this up.' I was then allocated to the nursing staff, that was fine for six months. The person for who I worked, she was great, she had been in touch with arthritis a great deal and she understood it and she was very very helpful but she retired and her successor is not so helpful so I wasn't finding that easy.

As with other spheres of daily existence what appear to be minor matters become significant problems in the context of disability such that small obstacles become major barriers to a trouble-free life. The slowness with which organizations react to these problems can seriously affect the quality of a disabled person's work experience.

Mrs A: I do feel sometimes life might have been made a little easier for me. . . . There have been a lot of problems I've had at times like getting switches moved, all sorts of *little* things that might have made life easier and might have made my job easier. I had to wait nine months for a plug for an electric typewriter and in the meantime use a manual one. That was very hard. With a little help it makes a terrific difference.

Clearly, many of the problems associated with work are manageable if colleagues and superiors are understanding, prepared to offer practical assistance, and prepared to be somewhat flexible. Such is the importance of the responses of others that this may be the key to remaining in work. When asked if she had experienced any problems when at work, Mrs X said 'Oh yes, but the girls were marvellous and so was the boss. Oh marvellous, they helped me a lot. If it hadn't been for the girls I couldn't have stayed at work.' Similarly, Mr F was able to carry on in his job long after he was unfit for building work: 'My mates were doing the biggest part of the work for me, you see, so you know, I was in a position where I was able to carry on whereas other people would have had to chuck it sooner. As I say, I had good friends and we all owned the company so I was able to carry on for, say, three or four years more than the average person.' Mrs W was helped considerably by being allowed to make minor adjustments to her working day.

Mrs W: In walking along I used to fall over in the street if I had to hurry. The firm were very kind to me, they let me clock in about ten minutes late to miss the crowd because anybody push me and I'd fall over. And they let me do that. I was supposed to make the time up at night time but they used to overlook that I used to go at the same time as anybody else.

By contrast, Mr P's immediate boss was not prepared to be flexible and insisted he do his share of relief work which involved walking from lift to lift and taking over while the operator went for a short break: 'I was in agony when I got home but he wouldn't let me off.' Eventually, Mr P went to his union representative, requested a transfer and was moved to a job in another government building.

Securing the help of colleagues and superiors does, of course, presuppose that the person is identified by others as disabled and in need of special consideration and means that they must be told of the presence of chronic illness and its attendant limitations. This is particularly the case where the illness is not immediately apparent to others. Consequently, Mrs A made a point of telling others at work that she did have certain problems.

> *Mrs A:* In a working situation I've found it better to tell people immediately that you have difficulty and then there isn't too much embarrassment. I have said 'Look, I am arthritic, I have weak wrists and I can't manage to do things,' and this has worked quite well. If you went into a job and tried to behave normally and gradually people realized you were handicapped this might create much more embarrassment.

However, revealing a disability may result in the person being categorized by others as helpless or even normally incompetent, and people may unwittingly step over the very fine dividing line between providing necessary help and degrading and unwanted attention. Mrs T was confined to a wheelchair and so could not help her disability being generally known. Moreover, she had to enlist the help of colleagues because she found it impossible to use the facilities at work. When she moved to her new job, she was on the receiving end of the wrong kind of help, and this was part of a series of events that gave rise to her decision to give up paid work.

> *Mrs T:* I didn't settle down in the job because strangely enough the people there were too kind to me and I began to feel a bit oppressed. The set-up there was such that I couldn't go for example to the Ladies on my own for the simple reason that the doors were in a heavy frame and they were much too hard for me to push open. So having discovered this and having obviously then had to ask somebody to come with me, which I didn't mind doing in the slightest don't think

that, word very quickly got round and so I was the faced with a situation that six or seven girls during the course of the morning or the afternoon would come and say 'Do you want to go to the Ladies?' Now this was extremely nice and something that I appreciated and I would obviously take up the option at least once in the morning and once in the afternoon but there was one woman there, she was older than I was and I think I possibly resented her because she was in much the same position as I was at my previous company, she was a charming woman but she got on my nerves. She would say to me things like, 'You're sure you've dried your hands properly?' and at the beginning I took this as a joke but after a while this really began to aggravate me.

Calling on the assistance of others in performing the work task is one of a set of alternative strategies which may be employed to cope with the problems associated with doing a particular job. One other is to negotiate an occupational role more easily managed with reduced physical capacities. After initially relying on his work mates, Mr F took over a set of essential but less demanding tasks.

Mr F: I never done any of the hard work, I done most of the running around, the driving around and collecting stuff, and things like that, just that. It saved other people from doing it, you know, at least I was being useful.

Although the company did business throughout England and the work involved travelling around the country, Mr F was allowed to handle the London end of the trade so as to reduce the necessity for him to be away from home.

Miss L, who joined the Civil Service because of their reputation for being flexible where disabled employees were involved, successfully negotiated her way through a succession of jobs until she found one which was suitable. Physical effort was difficult, and she wanted a position which involved little in the way of lifting or carrying.

Miss L: I had to give up one job, it was lugging great stacks of files. I said I would keep more well if I did something more in the line of brain work. They tried very hard to find me a job with not much physical work . . . you've got to do some 'cus I don't just like sitting all day, but it was pulling great boxes down this was the thing.

This strategy may be preferred by those who are unwilling to rely on the assistance and goodwill of their colleagues either because they wish to avoid being dependent or because they wish to conceal their illness.

Miss L: I don't want to say at work 'Can you do this? Would you mind doing that?' because it looks as if you're being, you know . . . 'cus I look fairly well, you see, I don't look ill and people say 'Well, what's wrong?' and though they may be helpful once or twice they get fed up with it if you keep asking. I've adjusted myself at home in the way I live but at work I don't want people to be aware that I've got rheumatoid arthritis, I don't want them to look on me as a poor little invalid.

In this way finding a job that can be managed without help solves a number of problems. As far as Miss L was concerned it meant she could remain in paid employment and protect her public identity by avoiding labels such as invalid. However, this strategy was not entirely free of symbolic loss. As she also remarked, 'I don't like saying I can't do a job.'

Where a job cannot be reorganized along less demanding lines and where the individual concerned refuses to be dependent upon the help and goodwill of others, then it may prove difficult to remain at work. Becoming unemployed may be a strategy which resolves the problematic aspects of work. For example, Mr I and the fiercely independent Mrs I both gave up their jobs soon after Mr I came out of hospital rather than be carried by others.

Mr I: I mean there were four or five blokes worked with me and they were carrying me like, you know, wouldn't let me bend down, wouldn't let me go up the stairs, wouldn't let me go on the grass if it was damp. . . .
Mrs I: I mean they couldn't keep on carrying you forever sometime they're going to get fed up doing it, ain't they?

Mrs I: When he was really getting, like his off days, I sort of phoned up my guv'nor and said 'I won't be in today Les's not well' and, er, next day he'd be a lot better and I'd go into work and then I was off the next when he got bad, you know. I was mucking him about, you know, he was very kind to me an' all this but I mean, as I say, they just can't go on forever doing it, you know, you can't keep on accepting his kindness all the time and I had to tell him 'It's no good me mucking you about.' I said 'You might as well get yourself another barmaid and cleaner, you know, I just can't come and work and that's it.' I didn't want to pack up work, I mean, I'd go to work if I could. I mean, the guy said I could go back to work any time I want but I know it won't be, it'll just be like before being carried again. You can't have people carrying you all the time.

Disadvantage in the labour market

Probably because the character of rheumatoid arthritis means that sufferers tend to leave the labour force never to return, the people interviewed here provided only limited data concerning disadvantage with respect to work. However, some of their accounts did illustrate some of the ways in which chronic illness and disability may create problems in terms of finding work, keeping work, and securing satisfactory careers.

None of the eight people recently unemployed and still wanting to work had yet tried their chances on the labour market. Most were waiting for a reduction in their levels of pain or more general improvements in their health before seeking to return to their previous jobs or looking for less demanding work. Consequently, they had yet to discover whether or not their disability was to prove a disadvantage in finding satisfactory employment or if it would prevent their returning to work altogether. Some, however, did expect to encounter difficulty in getting an employer to accept them.

> *Mrs A:* I keep wondering frankly, I don't know if I'd have much success in getting work now, I mean the situation is so bad isn't it and I think if you've got two people perhaps of my age who apply for a job and one has arthritis and the other doesn't I think you fairly reasonably take the other one, I think I would if I were an employer.

Mr M, who wanted to return to his job as Assistant General Manager to a local firm, had recently been sent to see their company doctor but had not been given their decision regarding his future. He was, however, pessimistic about the likelihood of his return and his long-term prospects.

> *Mr M:* I know for a fact the company don't want me back 'cus they told me so, they put it in the terms, well, there's three alternatives, one I've been there for over eight years so they owe me a certain amount of loyalty and feel they should give me something to do, secondly the other alternative was they would give me the sack, and the third alternative was they would sort of give me some money and say 'Goodbye, it's been nice knowing you.' I think they'll do everything in their power not to take me back.
>
> *Int:* What will happen if you don't go back to your old job?
>
> *Mr M:* I've given that a great deal of thought and to be honest with you I'd be absolutely scared stiff to see what happens next. If I do try and get back and they chuck me out I feel that I've got a handicap and I don't think people will take me. I'm going to be probably going to work, I'm going to have two or three good days and one day when I won't be able to go in and I used to employ and hire and fire people and you're running a production line and there's a bloke like me, there he's no flipping good to you at all.

The pessimism of Mrs A and Mr M regarding the likelihood of an employer taking them in preference to a non-disabled person was borne out in the accounts of some of the other people who had tried unsuccessfully to find jobs. These cases came close to what may be regarded as discrimination against the disabled worker. Mrs T had entered the labour force at the age of 22 as a result of a chance meeting with a friend's employer. Despite the fact that she had little in the way of formal education (she had a history of chronic illness stretching back to early childhood), 'he took a terrible risk and offered me a job there and then'. The job was in the accounts department of a small depot of a supplier of solid fuel, and after being promoted to manageress, she moved to a larger depot where she eventually became manageress again. After a short spell working at the company's head office, she left work and spent six months at home.

> *Mrs T:* After six months I began to get fidgety and tried to find myself another job. Now that was a very great mistake because for the first time in my life I was confronted by the labour market and this was the dreadful thing, people didn't tell me the truth. You see we used to get the local papers and I would ring about jobs and I'd give my age and my experience and in nearly every case it was the same, they would say, they were bending over backwards, 'Oh yes, Mrs T, why don't you come and see us?' implying that it was a mere formality that I went just to give them my insurance card. Well, I don't believe in taking advantage but the first time it was only an afterthought that I said 'Oh, I am sorry but it completely slipped my memory but I am disabled and in a wheelchair' and that was when the problems started. Quite suddenly there were all manner of reasons why I shouldn't be suitable. One that I was told on several occasions was that in view of my experience that quite obviously they wouldn't be able to give me the salary to which I was accustomed. Like a fool the first two or three times I argued, you know, I said that I didn't want to go to work for an enormous salary but I wanted to work and that I would pay for a car to take me backwards and forwards and as long as I covered that. I don't know whether they thought I was, maybe they did, thought I was some kind of nut that nobody wants, to go out to work to make at the end of it one pound or thirty bob maybe that was it.

One way of avoiding those kinds of difficulties, at least for those whose disability is either not too severe or not visible, is to conceal the presence of chronic illness.

> *Mrs D:* When I was at work before, people didn't know I had this, you know, it didn't come up in a conversation or anything 'cus they didn't even know I had it 'cus it didn't show. Even my boss didn't know I had a hip replacement, nobody knew. I just didn't bring it up, I didn't see why I should but now you can see the way I'm walking.

As many of the accounts in previous sections reveal, chronically sick people may experience a number of problems with regard to work, ranging from an inability to perform necessary tasks to overprotectiveness or discrimination on the part of employers or work mates. As far as people with rheumatoid arthritis are concerned, perhaps the most significant of these is the incompatibility of the disease and its effects with the demands of most types of labour. The limitations in physical capacity may make even the most basic requirements of a job problematic, let alone the special manual or other skills involved. For example, mobility around the place of work can be a major problem. Even so-called sedentary occupations such as routine clerical work require a degree of mobility around the work setting. Despite being capable of performing the work task itself, mobility problems may have consequences for the person's ability to remain employed. Mr P was asked to leave his job because of his limited mobility.

> *Mr P:* I took a job setting up at the Polytechnic but as I couldn't get around to the jobs they packed me in. You see you were on hand, on call, for all the students. If anything went wrong you'd be called in, and they said 'It's taking you too long to get to . . . and if one of them has an accident and it's time before you get there then. . . .' I was the only one and there was twenty-six lathes, four milling machines, one jig borer . . . each student would call you and then there was benches as well to help them out. The Principal called me up to his office and he said 'It's a case of, er, it's a hazard if you don't get there in time, and these students, they don't know nothing and if they do have trouble we'll be in trouble.' So they asked me to leave, so I did.

A second potentially problematic requirement of paid work is regular attendance and reasonably consistent time keeping. The fluctuating character of rheumatoid arthritis and the additional time needed to accomplish everyday activities may result in the person becoming an unreliable employee and lead to dismissal. In the early stages of Miss L's arthritis, before it had been diagnosed, it was taking her two hours or more to get up in the morning and get into work. Finally, she was told that because she kept coming in so late they were unable to keep her on. As Miss L commented, 'You couldn't blame them really.' Subsequently, she found herself a clerical job with the Civil Service where she knew disabled people were well treated and where erratic performance and periods of sick leave were accommodated: 'I don't have to worry too much if I get a flare-up, knowing they realize I have a problem.'

Even where chronic illness and disability do not prevent a person finding work or remaining within the workforce, it may have a significant impact on career development and the attainment of more satisfying and highly rewarded jobs. It may prevent entry into desired occupations or restrict the chances of promotion within them. Disabled since childhood, Mrs T found her career choices to be very limited.

Mrs T: I started off as a child as most girls do wanting to be a hairdresser but as soon as I got some sense into my head I desperately wanted to be a research scientist but when I started coming near to . . . when I was in hospital, [at age 15] I realized that I was going to be pretty severely handicapped and together with the fact that I had virtually no education anyway I realized that the chances of anyone accepting me were very slim and I was in a bit of a limbo about that time not being sure what I could do, knowing I would never be able to type, not satisfactorily to earn my living, because I'd never be able to type fast enough. So really, book-keeping was at that time really the only thing open to me because I had to have a job where I did a lot of sitting down. I've never ceased to regret that I couldn't have done something more positive.

Mrs A and Miss L had been in secretarial and clerical positions and both discovered that their opportunities had been adversely affected, although in somewhat different ways. Mrs A had been a secretary in a government department for 38 years and had been promoted to a senior position before her arthritis began to have any real effect on her work. For the last five years her condition had been deteriorating, and she had taken increasing amounts of sick leave. This she felt had had some influence on the kinds of jobs she had been given.

Mrs A: I'd no ambition to go higher than Senior Secretary, this is the top secretarial post in the department, and I really wasn't trained for anything but secretarial work so I don't think I could have gone any higher. I haven't been passed over or anything like that . . . it's just that in you're own grade you don't do quite so well. You see, when you get a reputation for a great deal of sick leave you're not so easy to place and you find that you're not getting a job you're capable of doing. I suppose this is understandable but it's jolly hard sometimes.

Miss L had been a secretary prior to onset but difficulty in typing meant that she was now restricted to clerical work. In the organization in which she worked the salary differentials between secretarial and clerical staff were not great. However, there was a difference in status such that the latter were not as well regarded as the former: 'You're just a clerk here.' While the salary she received was very good for a clerical position, the job itself was 'not too exciting' and she had thought of seeking promotion and a more challenging job.

Miss L: One part of me would like to get on and apply for a higher position, another part says I might do that and have another flare-up. There I'd be in a higher position with more responsibility and it's annoying if people don't turn up or aren't there half the time. People, however generous they are they still you've got to be there and cover a job, haven't you? So half of me is quite ambitious really. I'd like to. . . . I mean, I think I can do something better. I mean, my mind says I could do something a lot more but I think it would be worrying to me thinking I'm all right for a long time and then something happens.

For both of these women the limitations in career opportunities they experienced were rooted in the uncertain course of rheumatoid arthritis and their inability to guarantee consistent attendance at work. They saw themselves as actually or potentially unreliable workers or believed they were seen as such by others. Consequently, Miss L chose to remain in a low status job where absences might be more easily managed by her employers rather than seek a more senior post where sick leave would result in more disruption for the organization. A sense of obligation to others coupled with an unwillingness to test the limits of their tolerance meant that her career potential remained unexplored. In return she gained relative peace of mind. Having twisted her knee she had three months off work:

> *Miss L:* That's a long time to be away from a job, isn't it? And if it's a job somebody else can do somebody can cover you or, if it's not so important, you don't feel so worried about it, do you?

The decision to give up work

As some of the data presented above indicates, not wanting to be dependent upon others is only one of the reasons the respondents gave for deciding to stop working. For some, the decision was clear cut; their arthritis became so severe they were no longer able to get to work or do the job. Mrs K had to leave her job in a grocery store because she was unable to reach up to take things off shelves, and Mr E abandoned work when the effort of getting there became too much.

> *Mr E:* That was a struggle after a time I can tell you . . . I used to have to walk up this hill here to the office to sign on every morning and at the finish I just couldn't get up there. I was hanging onto that railing up there pulling myself up.

For others, the job had been manageable despite pain and limited mobility and they finally gave up work following pressure from doctors and employers and a careful assessment of the gains and losses.

A good example of the latter is the case of Mrs A. At the first interview she was on sick leave and at that time her biggest problem was deciding whether to retire or to return to work. One factor in favour of her giving up her job was the worry associated with her increasing inability to get through the work.

Mrs A: It was taking me longer to do the work and also I felt I wasn't doing all those things . . . this sounds terribly big-headed but I'm a good secretary and there are lots of jobs you do which aren't in the rule book and I found I wasn't getting time to do those because it was taking me all my time to do routine work. Well, that takes a lot of the joy out of the job.

While she thought that it would be advisable to stop working for the beneficial effect of rest on her arthritis, other factors needed to be taken into account. Given that she was the main provider, giving up work would involve a considerable financial loss.

Mrs A: There is the financial situation . . . I don't know if my husband is ever going to work again, I doubt it personally but . . . I just don't know . . . would I be more worried at home with less to do and perhaps more financial problems or would I find eventually I couldn't continue with work and I've got myself into a much worse state by that time and was far worse off? I just don't know . . . as I said, I'm still thinking.

By the time of the second interview one year later, Mrs A had stopped working. Because she had taken one year's sick leave in the previous four her employers contacted her GP and consultant, and between them it was decided that she would be retired.

As Mrs A had anticipated, the financial loss sustained through giving up work was quite considerable and in the face of increasing difficulty she began to consider making the effort of returning to work. She was persuaded by her doctor that the only way in which her arthritis would improve was if she led a much quieter life, and she agreed. The problematic aspects of continuing to work were then replaced by the problem of managing a satisfactory existence with a much reduced income.

Such pressure by doctors or others did not seem to give rise to much resentment on the part of the persons concerned where it helped to resolve their own ambiguity about remaining at work, where it was seen to be in their own best interests, or where they accepted their own limitations as employees. Mr H said, commenting on his employer's desire to see him leave work, 'I was having a bad time and obviously the firm is not there as a charity, they're there to run a business, you know, so I can understand.'

One option considered by some of the respondents wanting to resume work was to go back to their previous job. Because they expected to encounter a number of problems in their attempts to manage work, returning to familiar tasks offered a number of key advantages.

Mr M: I'd sooner go back to the devil I know rather than try something completely new. I know the job, I can probably handle it with the difficulties I've got. I'd rather go back to the firm although they're not treating me very well I'd rather go back there and sort the problems out there.

Int: Do you foresee any difficulties if you do go back?

Mr M: I would think so but if I go back to an environment I know I may be able to find ways of solving these problems, erm . . . 'cus I know where the machinery is . . . I don't know what problems will arise . . . I won't know until I go back.

Mr F had tried to return to his former job but this did little more than reaffirm that he was unfit for that kind of work. Consequently, he was forced to pursue a number of alternatives.

Mr F: I can't go back to the sites 'cus I'm more a liability there than anything else. I have tried, you know, going back and doing bits and pieces but I'm just an embarrassment 'cus it's mostly machinery they handle and building work. I prefer to keep out of the way 'cus if they drop a machine on me I'd be worse off. I was hoping to get a job across the road here with this firm and I was talking to the guv'nor. I spoke to him earlier in the year but they went to an exhibition over in Germany and never sold a thing so he's just let off 14 people, so that's gone through. I'm just going to wait now and get out of London completely, that's about all I'm waiting for.

Some of the women were thinking about trying part-time work, in the hope that it would not over burden their limited personal resources. Mrs A said 'Then I would set out in the morning and think "Well, this is fine, I *know* I can get through it." ' Despite some improvement since she stopped working, she was still unable to lift and carry or reach above her head. Thinking about the kinds of jobs she might be able to do, she said 'I just don't know what's the answer.' For Mrs I, a return to work would only be possible once the family had moved house and acquired the aids and adaptations to enable her disabled husband to cope alone at home.

Mrs I: You know, I just want to get out to see what equipment they're going to put in the new flat to see how helpful it is 'cus if it's helpful, you know, and he says 'well, you can try and get a little job for a couple of hours.' I'd like to work for a couple of hours as long as I know he's all right but, I mean, no way can I go while we're here. If I can get a little job once I know all the fitments are there and he's going to manage that I shall feel at ease even if it's only a couple of hours at work. Most likely I'll go back to bar work eleven till three like, do lunch times, but I wouldn't do it now, I couldn't go back to work now.

Int: Would it worry you?

Mrs I: Yes, yes, I mean the children being at school all day and him being left on his own and if I have to go out before he gets up and I don't know how he feels if he gets a bad morning and can't get out of bed he's stuck there till I get home that's the way it'd be. If he had this equipment to help him get about I'd feel easier in myself and most likely could get a job even if it's only for a couple of hours it'd be something.

While Mr F believed a better future would be attained by moving out of London, the I's believed that specially adapted housing would begin to restore their independence and allow them to go someway towards reconstructing their family life.

The meaning of work

The meaning and significance of work and the centrality of work in everyday life are perhaps perceived most acutely by the unemployed. Once lost, what may have been the tedium of a nine-to-five job involving repetition and routine becomes an activity that gave structure and purpose to everyday existence. For both the disabled and non-disabled, becoming unemployed involves much more than a loss of income. In fact, the non-financial losses sustained may be more important than the sudden reduction in earnings that follows giving up work. Of course, the meaning of ceasing to work varies with individual circumstances. Its consequences are likely to be different for a single man living alone than for a married woman with a husband who is in paid work, and the impact on the family is likely to differ according to whether it is the main, rather than an associate, breadwinner who becomes disabled and unfit for work. Its effects may also vary when seen in the context of individual motives and the availability of viable alternative activities. Whatever the consequences, all of those who had given up paid work expressed some regret at losing their job.

The significance of work and its place within everyday life are perhaps best illustrated by the case of Mr M. He was single, lived alone, and had left his job one year before he was first interviewed. At the time of the first interview he was uncertain whether or not his firm would take him back nor was he sure that he was capable of going back to full-time work. Since the latter problem had more serious long-term implications, he was very anxious to go back to his old job in order to resolve the uncertainty. He was very hostile towards all those dealing with his case, whom he believed were unhelpful and failing to provide him with the means to deal with the problem.

Mr M: I don't enjoy sitting down here 24 hours a day feeling sorry for myself. If I can get answers to questions, if I can get back moving, I've got, in my own mind, to find out if I can go back to work or not, so the only way is to go back and find out and if I can't do it then I've bloody well had it. I've got to go on a completely different track and have a different attitude towards life, you know. I mean, this doctor I went to he says 'What's your attitude about going back to work?' I said 'Look, we either go for broke. It's as simple as that. I either do it or I can't do it and then that's a problem we've got to face.' I mean, sitting down on my backside all day long doing nothing, just getting angry with everyone around me isn't going to solve my problem at all, is it? I've got to satisfy myself if I can do it or I can't.

Mr M's frustration arose from the feeling that little was being done either to improve his condition medically or to clarify the uncertainty regarding his prospects of returning to work. Clearly, he was at a crucial point in his career. If he was able to return to work the structure of his life would remain largely intact, if not, both his actions and his attitudes had to be adjusted accordingly. Until that dilemma was resolved there appeared little he could do to help himself and little point in beginning to reorganize his life in the pursuit of new objectives.

In talking about their work the respondents discussed the benefits they derived from being in paid employment and the problems they experienced on giving up their jobs. The women experienced job loss as acutely as the men and few were content to settle into the role of housewife. Contrary to expectations, the men tended to talk about boredom, loneliness, and the frustration of being confined to the house while the women talked about the additional problems of independence, identity, achievement, and involvement. Both, however, reported being depressed and miserable on giving up work.

Mr I and Mr F had jobs which took them out and about and brought them into contact with many other people. Mr I had been caretaker of the block of flats in which he and his family still lived, where his duties had included general maintenance and dealing with the many problems brought to him by the other tenants: 'I was always busy, always about, always on my feet, I was always out in the fresh air, never sat indoors.' Mr F's job had involved installing and servicing launderettes: 'I was out meeting people all the time, during the day people were always coming and going, you know. You had a joke and mucked about.' Consequently, giving up work transformed their existence, and both found staying at home hard to bear. Mrs I, commenting on her husband, said 'If it's a nice day he sits on a stool by the door but that's not out really, is it? It's just at the door. As I say, at first he was very miserable, he's never been out of work. He was unbearable at first but he's had to learn to accept it, he can't go out working and that's it.' Mr F said 'To come down here in the morning and to stay here all day, that used to get me.'

Even routine office work offered similar benefits and contrasted sharply with the experience of being out of a job.

> *Mrs N:* I didn't want to stop work but it helped . . . but after being used, you know, you get used to all the people in the office, you know, you have your laughs and your jokes and you're seeing people everyday, then all of a sudden I was thrown back home and stuck indoors just sitting there on my own.

In addition to loneliness Mr P found the lack of something to do a major problem.

> *Mr P:* I get so bored here, you know, since giving up I didn't know what to do and, er, get so bored. . . . It upsets me a lot, I always liked doing something with me hands, you know, er, in the flat you can't do much. It's much better to keep yourself busy.

As the next section will demonstrate, the monetary rewards derived from work are not insignificant; poverty is an important consequence of job loss. However, money does not only mean a decent standard of living, it also means independence, freeing an individual from reliance upon the support of others. Mrs D and Mrs N both missed having their own money after they gave up work, Mrs N because she was no longer able to indulge her children and grandchildren: 'I used to get a great deal of pleasure out of that which I miss now because I don't have my own money to do it.' For Miss L, however, being in work and earning her own living was the key to her domestic harmony and her peace of mind. After living in a bed-sitter for a number of years, she decided to return to live in her sister's house where they would share expenses.

> *Miss L:* If you're living with somebody, if you have a job you're paying your way, you're not dependent upon anybody or . . . this is what I like to feel, that I've got enough money not to be dependent. You don't have to live on other people's generosity.

She was unable to do any but the lightest housework, but this did not mean it became the responsibility of her sister.

> *Miss L:* This is why, being independent, I can pay half towards a cleaner. I don't have to think I can't do the cleaning . . . my sister, she has quite a hard job, and I can't expect her to come home and start cleaning and clean my room and things so, erm, this is the thing, money makes you independent. I can afford to pay for a lady to come in and do the jobs.

In this way money provides for easy solutions to some of the practical problems of everyday living and, coincidentally, modifies the relationships between disabled persons and others. Because of the significance of work in the context of Miss L's life, she organized herself in a manner to maximize her chances of being able to continue in her job. She restricted herself to going out no more than twice a week: 'I could go out more really but if I want to keep working I feel I've got to live a fairly steady life. It sounds a bit boring, I know.'

For some, staying in paid work was a means of pursuing the more general strategy of 'carrying on'. By refusing to give in and adopt a more limited lifestyle, they attempted to minimize the impact of their illness and thereby avoid accepting a disabled status. For Mrs N remaining active and remaining in work was the way to prevent her condition from transforming her into a crippled person.

> *Mrs N:* When I first had it I still carried on work because I was under the impression that if you let it go you get, you know, sort of set and you wouldn't be able to move. I thought 'No, I'm not going to let it get on top of me, I'll push on and on.' I was dragging myself to work, absolutely dragging myself and I thought, 'No, I won't give in!' because I was under the impression you mustn't give way to these things, you keep going, you know, stop the joints seizing up 'cus that's how I imagined you became crippled, through letting it get a hold.

Similarly, Mrs V carried on working as a waitress despite earning low wages and suffering as a result.

> *Mrs V:* I used to come home from work crying I was in so much pain but I still done it, I really still done it. It wasn't for the money so much, three pounds ten shillings I used to get there, it was to make me keep myself going.

While work provides an opportunity for keeping going and refusing to succumb to pain and discomfort, it also provides an essential motive for so doing. Many of the respondents described how easy it would have been some days to have given in to pain and stayed in bed rather than face the effort of getting up and getting dressed. Even though this was seen as the start of a downward drift into helplessness and total disability, it was sometimes difficult to avoid. Having something to get up and get going for provided an added incentive for fighting these undesirable feelings of wanting to give up. Mrs R emphasized the importance of having some responsibility to fulfil. She began doing voluntary work after she had been asked by her consultant to run a stall for the disabled at an exhibition in London: 'It meant that I had to get out. I had to drive and it gave me a certain amount of independence.' Subsequently, she opened a charity shop which she ran with the help of her daughter.

> *Mrs R:* When we had this shop I used to make myself go, this was a very good thing it kept me going. I thought 'Now, if I don't get there

the shop isn't going to open and there will be people outside waiting.' Everyone with this complaint should have something, not that they can go to when they please, but they've got a commitment like with this shop. Some days I'd feel like nothing on earth but I knew I'd got to be there and it made me get going.

In this way, having a commitment and having others dependent upon one's efforts gives meaning to the painful and protracted struggle of coping with the effects of rheumatoid arthritis. Even so, those without paid or voluntary work or other such activity generally invested time and energy in getting out of bed, washing, and dressing. These became valued in themselves, despite the fact that they might lead to a little more than sitting alone at home.

As Morse and Weiss (1955) have suggested, work ties an individual into the wider society and gives a sense of purpose in life. It also provides the opportunity to accomplish things and to contribute to the general good. As such it is an important source of identity. This is applicable to both the disabled and non-disabled, of both domestic and paid work, and of managerial and non-managerial positions. Mrs A, for example, talked of the sense of achievement she derived from her job as a secretary: 'You had a very definite feeling of being part of a large organization and a job well done and at the end of the day you came home and felt it was all worthwhile.'

Where a person finds work after becoming chronically ill, the ability to do a job, no matter how menial or poorly paid, may create an even greater sense of accomplishment in the world and contribute to the construction of identity. Mrs T began work at the age of 22 much against the wishes of her parents who wanted her to have a year's convalescence following a series of operations.

> *Int:* You were quite keen to start work were you?
> *Mrs T:* I was bending over backwards, bending over backwards and nobody was more proud of me than me when I came home with my first wage packet. I remember I was two weeks short of 22 when I started work and I came home with my wage packet of three pounds. It wasn't much but I thought that was marvellous.

While the disabled and non-disabled unemployed may have problems in common, there are differences between their respective situations. Although both may interpret the advent of unemployment as evidence of personal failure, the latter at least have access to alternative explanations which may help to preserve their identity. They may, for example, point to government policy or world recession to account for their lack of a job. Because we rarely question the organization of work at the everyday level, it is not unreasonable to suppose that the disabled see their exclusion from the labour force as the result of their own inadequacy. For them unemployment robs them of a sense of achievement and a sense of self: because it is readily seen as the result of physical incapacity it is tied exclusively to them.

Mrs A: I didn't mind (giving up work) at the time but I've got a bit neurotic about it since. You have the feeling of a job undone, of having broken off, you know, before you completed something. You tend to feel, what's the expression for this? a little bit second class, not able to keep up with the general run of things. Oh, I got very neurotic about it a little while ago and my husband had to put up with a great deal in the way of tears and misery but I'm trying hard not to feel that way because there's lots I can do. I'd still like to be able to do work of some kind, you know, I get a bit broody over that at times.

Mrs A's comment about not being able to keep up with the general run of things was echoed by Mr K in talking about his wife's disability.

Mr K: I think it's had a very bad effect on her mentally because, er, always having worked hard all her life and brought up a family and always being sort of at the centre of everything and being able to do the washing and the ironing and the cooking and to suddenly, to suddenly get cut down like this I think it has a great disturbing effect mentally.

Mrs K had worked following her marriage and continued to work while bringing up five children. For such people the inability to do a job or continue doing housework creates boredom and frustration. They become socially marginal, no longer centrally involved in everyday affairs but confined to the periphery as a mere observer of the activities of others. As with some of the men interviewed by Morse and Weiss (1955), a life without work is a life without activity and a life with nothing to do. Even the mundane tasks of household management cannot be used to keep occupied.

Mrs K: I mean, now I sit here and say to my husband, 'Oh, I wish I could do this, I wish I could do that.' He says 'You sit down,' you know, and sometimes I'd think to myself 'I'd love to do that but I can't.'

Obviously, the advent of unemployment in one individual, whatever its origin, is going to have some consequences for other members of the family. At the very least these others may have to tolerate and manage the distress and frustration of the person concerned or their standard of living may be reduced by the inability of that person to secure an adequate income. It is not necessarily the case that the effect on others is invariably

negative, and the onset of unemployment may be viewed quite differently by the unemployed and their spouses. Some men, for example, were
quite keen for their wives to stop work. Mrs A's husband was a patient at
a psychiatric day hospital and had not worked himself for a number of
years. He was quite prepared to put up with the financial consequences of
her leaving her job because that would restore the equality of their
relationship.

> *Mrs A:* He's all for it, one hundred per cent. He feels very badly that
> he's, you know, that I'm the sole provider, but this is something that
> can't be helped and he is very much all for it. His attitude is, 'Well, if we
> can't manage we'll have to go to Social Security and see what they can
> do.'

Mrs W's husband demanded that she give up work, perhaps to restore
his public image as an adequate provider for his family.

> *Mrs W:* My husband got very angry with me. He said he didn't need
> me to go to work and it was stupid and people were thinking 'God, that
> poor woman struggling to work' and he said 'You'll just have to give it
> up' and that, and I didn't really want to leave 'cus I had such a good
> position. When you've worked a long time like that and you've got a
> good position it's hard to give it up but I did.

In both of these instances the meaning of unemployment was quite
different for the women and their husbands. Their attempts to remain in
the labour force constituted a greater threat to the identity and status of
the men involved than the financial loss sustained by their having no job.
As always, the activities of our close associates reflect upon our self image
and public character.

Alternatives to work

Those who were unable to work were often faced with the problem of
what to do with their time. This seemed to be particularly so for the men
and those who lived alone. In fact, the single men living alone had few
resources other than work to occupy their time and give purpose and
structure to their day. The women more frequently immersed themselves
in family life and domestic roles, and those who lived with others also
seemed to have wider kin and friendship networks which could be called
upon to help fill surplus time. Where married women were not able or not
allowed by others to resort to a domestic role, they too were left with the
boredom and frustration of little to do. It was those with no means of
filling their time who were the unhappiest and most desperate for
alternatives to work.

Some of the women escaped boredom and loneliness by becoming involved in activities outside the home; like Mrs R and Mrs W who did voluntary and political work and Mrs A who found the local church a rich source of activities and social contacts. Their days were always busy, taken up by telephone calls and people who dropped in in connection with this work. The men seemed to find it more difficult to develop substitute activities and either stayed at home, passing the time as best they could, or made use of day centres for the disabled. For Mr P and Mr C, both single men living alone, day centres were their sole sources of activity and social contact. However, day centres were not a solution to all those needing stimulation and outside interests. Mr I had been to see his local day centre but found it to be full of severely disabled people and was advised by the manager not to go. His rehabilitation officer was trying to organize some work at home just to give him something to occupy his mind. Mrs D, the only woman to go to a centre, said 'I'd feel happier if I was working in a normal atmosphere where there wasn't a lot of disabled people', so found it inappropriate to her needs. Even those who enjoyed the contacts and activity these centres offered found them to be only a partial answer to their problem. Space or transportation were sometimes in short supply and they were only able to go for two days per week, or pain and immobility sometimes meant that they had to stay at home for days on end. As a consequence, they might see no one and do nothing. When Mr P talked about the days he was unable to get to the day centre, I asked if he got bored:

> *Mr P:* Oh I go nuts, I go really barmy, sometimes I don't know what to do with myself. I want to go out, I want to do things but I can't. I suppose when I don't go to the centre I get lonesome, it's lonesomeness I think. When I could do things it didn't bother me, I could find something to do in the place to mess about with. Now I can't do it, I know I can't. All you've got is the television. You try and sleep, you try and sleep the time away, I seem to be doing more sleeping lately to try and sleep it off.

Income

While unemployment has a number of undesirable effects, one of its more immediate and readily apparent consequences is a reduction in income and a decline in standards of living. The loss of physical resources that stems from chronic disease almost invariably leads to a loss of material resources in the form of money and wealth. It should come as no surprise then to find that all studies of long-term sickness or poverty have found a correlation between the two. It could be argued that disabled people who receive a low income are more disadvantaged than the able-bodied poor if only because disability creates extra needs and entails extra expense (Walker 1981). Consequently, a limited income has to be spread that much further. For example, the disabled may need to spend more on heating, special clothing, and diets, or they may need to replace clothing and furniture more frequently because of damage caused by wheelchairs and other aids (Hyman 1977; Harris 1971). Perhaps a more important source of disadvantage is this: the reduced financial resources at the disposal of disabled people need to be spent in ways which compensate for their reduced capacity to perform the mundane practical tasks of everyday life. They may have to spend money to ensure that the house is cleaned and the shopping done, and because public transport is impossible even for those denied the mobility allowance, cars must be hired in order to undertake essential journeys such as visits to hospital. As Mrs I remarked at one interview, 'It's all money, isn't it?' Whether disabled or not, money is essential to achieve participation in the life of the community. For disabled people whose incomes often barely cover the basic essentials of living, there is nothing left over to pay for a fuller and more satisfying existence. It is the lack of money as much as the illness and its effects which prevents them from pursuing and attaining the good things in life. It is for these reasons that disabled people need more rather than less in the way of financial support.

The majority of those unable to work had experienced a substantial drop in income on giving up work. Mrs A's Civil Service pension and benefits combined totalled approximately half of her income while in work, Mr M's income had fallen from £80 per week to £23.65, and when Mr K gave up work to look after his disabled wife their income declined from £89 per week to £46. However, the extent to which these drops in income produced problems for the disabled person was very much a function of individual circumstance. Among this group of people those experiencing extreme hardship almost always lived alone. These were the people wholly dependent upon state benefits, either National Insurance payments or Supplementary Benefit, with no additional sources of income, who had to maintain a household without the aid of others. This is not to say that all those living alone were in financial difficulty even if dependent upon state support. Those with close family ties or extensive social networks seemed less likely to be or perhaps less likely to feel themselves to be living in poverty. Also experiencing hardship were those families with dependent children where the husband was disabled and the wife did not work.

Managing on a limited income

Quite simply, the problem confronting disabled people living on a small income is that of paying for the basic necessities of life and the extra needs created by the illness and its effects. Some of the people in this group managed to get by as a result of a number of strategies designed to maximize income or reduce expenditure. When these strategies were exhausted they had no option but to cope even if that meant doing without some of the basic necessities of life. Mrs V, who had £19 per week on which to live after her rent had been paid, said 'That's for everything. I manage on that. I've got to, there's nothing else.' For others, none of the strategies they employed were successful in making their income meet their outgoings and here life-long principles were abandoned and they accepted the accumulation of debt.

Getting into debt usually happened following a crisis such as the appearance of a large bill for a major item like gas, electricity, or the telephone, which could only be paid if other major items such as the rent were ignored. Since these represented recurring expenses, once in debt there seemed to be no way out. As Mr M pointed out when discussing his financial problems, his bills were the same now that he was existing on £23 per week as they had been when he had earned almost four times that amount. The only difference was that he now received a rent and rate rebate totalling £9 per week. This reduced the costs of his accommodation by half but still left only £13 a week to provide for all his other needs. Consequently, paying bills was difficult if not impossible and debt almost inevitable. As he said, 'Out of £23 a week you don't even break even, you're always juggling the figures around to try and manage.'

Small incomes require stringent financial planning if they are to be made to cover basic and other expenses. Over time some of the people interviewed developed routines for managing their everyday affairs and made sure that money was put by to pay the bills for major items of expenditure. Mr S was one of the better off disabled men receiving a War Disability Pension and other benefits but could 'just get by with it' only by careful allocation of available resources.

Mr S: We've got ourselves into a system now. We manage but we can't go mad. When you've got a wife that's got a good system like, you know, puts this up, that up, so much a day she's always done and she's sort of used to doing it, you know.

Mrs X put by a little money each week to pay her heating bills, and Mr P split his income in two, saving his small Civil Service pension and using his Invalidity Benefit to meet his other needs.

Mr P: I use an awful lot of heat in the winter 'cus I feel the cold very bad. I don't know what I'm going to do this year with electricity going up but I usually save enough. I put my pension in the Post Office and that's what I use that for. I don't touch it at all, I use it for that purpose, only the heating bills. The last one was £149. It comes in such a whack when you look at your savings you find you've barely got that amount to keep yourself viable, you have to ask if you can split it over two months, you know, it's difficult to pay that amount.

While arranging to pay large bills in instalments is one way of meeting heavy demands, it can lead to the accumulation of debt. When Mr and Mrs I were about to have their gas supply cut off because they were unable to pay a £70 bill, the Social Services department interceded on their behalf and it was agreed the bill would be paid off at £5 per week. As Mrs I said, 'I have been paying it but I've had the next gas bill in since then so I shall be like this all the time, just paying that £5 all the time. I mean even that is a struggle, it's just a big lump out of your money each time.'

Mr F managed his family finances by drawing on savings to supplement his Invalidity Benefit and his wife's wages. This also required a degree of forward planning: 'I've got it down to a fine art now that I only draw so much a week to make up a living wage on . . . it isn't dwindling away as fast as I thought it would and if there's anything left over it goes back to the bank and we keep it balanced that way.' Many others in this group had been forced to draw on savings either to buy essential equipment such as orthopaedic beds or to meet everyday living costs, but as a finite resource and one that could no longer be replenished they sometimes rapidly disappeared. Mr M's savings had been used within one year of his giving up work: 'All my savings have gone, I'm in trouble with the bank. I forget how much I owe them. Everything's gone, there's nothing left at all. I can't even afford to buy a pair of underpants or nothing.' However, not all of the people had savings to buffer the sudden decline in their income, and they found it particularly hard to manage in the initial stages of disability. Prior to becoming disabled Mr I and his wife had lived 'from day to day', finding temporary part-time work or saving hard over short periods of time in order to acquire household appliances or pay for holidays. With three young children, they had not been able to put anything by. Consequently, much needed items like a special bed had to be purchased out of their much reduced weekly income since their prior system of managing money was no longer viable.

Savings constitute one type of resource that may be employed to compensate for a drop in earning capacity. Some of the people were able to make use of other resources to reduce their basic expenses and live within the confines of their small incomes. For example, Mrs X avoided large heating bills by spending much of the winter quarter staying with her family. She had four daughters living away from home and would stay for two or three weeks with each: 'That's my family's way of saying "Come on, mum, we don't want any heating or fuel bills." ' Even so, the necessity to keep warm for the remainder of the year meant that spending on gas and electricity remained substantial. When not staying with her family, Mrs X went to a local luncheon club where she was able to get a good meal for as little as 10 pence: 'It makes all the difference. If I had to buy a meat meal as well as tea I couldn't manage.' Because her midweek spending on food was kept fairly low, she used some of what was saved to 'get that little bit extra at the weekend'. Similarly, Mr and Mrs K were unable to afford to buy meat and had lunch at a local day centre three or four times a week even though Mr K found little value in what they received: 'It's just something to eat, there's no body in it, I feel our diet would be a lot better if we could afford better things.'

Careful budgeting and the use of supplementary resources did not in and of themselves entirely solve the financial difficulties of this group of people. In all cases, the matching of income and expenditure meant some reduction in the amount of goods and services they consumed. The basic necessities of life, so-called luxuries, and social activities were all curtailed in the effort to keep within available resources and avoid going into debt. Consequently, these people were continually forced to make choices as to how their money was to be spent. In some cases the choices were very stark indeed, between buying food or paying bills:

Mrs V: I'd hate the bills to come in and have nothing to pay them with, that would worry me more than anything on earth so I just ease up on the groceries as much as I can.

One of the things most readily given up in the face of adverse financial circumstances were recreational and social activities, whether these be cultural events like trips to the theatre or simple pleasures like joining friends for a drink. While the physical difficulties of gaining access to social settings are important, the need to cut down on expenditure was also a significant barrier preventing these people from making full use of opportunities once enjoyed. For Mrs R, confined to a wheelchair and virtually housebound, going to the theatre was one of the joys of her existence. Because of the need to take the wheelchair, they always had to sit in the most expensive sectors of the theatre and were unable to take advantage of cheaper seats which were only reached by several flights of stairs. Even though Mrs R's husband was in work and earning a relatively substantial salary, they had had to cut back on their trips to see plays. Though this was very much regretted Mrs R saw it as part of a more general process affecting the disabled and non-disabled alike. In times of economic crisis, everybody had to limit spending in some way. Probably because it is not so readily interpreted as part of a wider trend but indicative of a slide into personal poverty, having to give up simpler but taken-for-granted activities sometimes had more impact.

Mr F: I think this is the biggest trouble, you know, with anybody that's been working all their life, that when they do finish, you know. . . . I used to like a few pints of beer, and that, and cigarettes and I used to back a horse but I've cut all that out. I just have a cigarette now. Even if I go out I seldom have a drink. If I want a drink I have a glass of something at home.

Mr and Mrs I found it very difficult to accept that they could no longer afford to go away on holiday. By saving throughout the year they had always managed to get away, and the year before Mr I became disabled they had been able to stay in a hotel. Their last holiday had been two years ago just after Mr I came out of hospital: 'The only reason we got that was we had friends in the Isle of Wight put us up.' Mrs I continued 'I used to look forward to my holiday. When the time comes I get the right hump, everybody going away and I don't go.' Their rehabilitation officer had mentioned the possibility that a holiday might be arranged through the local Social Services Department, and the I's were going to follow this up primarily for the benefit of their children.

Mrs I: I'd like to if only so the kids get away. I mean they could go away with the school but I just haven't the money to do it. My daughter wanted to go to Guernsey, it was £51, I said 'You just can't go.' They're all good kids, they don't deserve it, they need a holiday and that's it. My brother-in-law might take them down to his caravan for a couple of days but there again it's not a holiday is it, it's just for a couple of days.

That these were problems to which the I family were unaccustomed was underlined by Mr I at the close of this discussion: 'As I say, before I was like this we had none of this trouble, none at all.'

Cutting down on or cutting out altogether social and recreational activities, though necessary, rarely involved major savings. As financial hardship increased other cuts were considered which it was anticipated would make more contribution to the struggle to survive within a limited budget. Prime targets for such cuts were expensive aids such as telephones and cars. These were seen as a last resort because they were essential, facilitating other important activities like maintaining social contacts and mobility around the community. At the same time they were targets because they were expendable; in their absence the people concerned would have to adapt to a restricted and less satisfying life-style. Telephones were particularly useful to people who lived alone, so much so that Mrs V said 'I daren't be without that.' Mr M, however, did think he might have to lose his, despite its value, as he had been denied financial assistance with the rental and the bills.

Mr M: The telephone will have to go eventually and I would hate to lose that as that is my only contact with. . . . As I live on my own that is my only contact with anybody at all outside if I want anything, you know. I'd hate to lose it as it is so useful. It's an essential thing in my position. I cannot get help with the telephone as I'm not half dead. If you're half dead you'll get the grant on the telephone . . . and yet I could have an accident here quite easily . . . I could be carrying a pot of tea or anything like that and set it over me. There's all sorts of things could happen. It's different if there are two of you in a flat but if you're on your own that telephone is vital.

All of the people interviewed had some problem with mobility around the community, although this was conspicuously less consequential for those who had access to a car. Private transport significantly increased the range of places these disabled people could get to and the breadth of activities in which they were able to participate. They were expensive items, however, and some found cars too expensive to run and maintain.

While efforts to reduce consumption often meant that a small income did cover the basic necessities of life, some of the people interviewed found such poverty to be unacceptable. As a result, time and energy were also invested in the attempt to maximize personal or family income. Part-time work was considered by some or the spouse of some but rejected on the grounds that additional earnings would reduce welfare payments.

Mrs I: As soon as the Social know you're working, down it comes, more money off, so it's no benefit.

The only alternative was to seek additional state benefits such as the mobility allowance, attendance allowance, or invalid care allowance or to apply for discretionary payments to supplement benefits already received. These extra resources were sought in order that money currently spent on basic needs could be freed for use elsewhere. Mrs I had applied for the invalid care allowance which would have added £18 a week to the family income: 'I mean £18 that would have been my food money', and Mr M had applied for a heating allowance: '£1.80 a week that would contribute towards leaving a few bob for you to do something else.' In applying for these payments, Mrs I and Mr M became confronted with what they came to perceive as a complex and fundamentally unjust system of financial provision (see Chapter 7).

The difficulty disabled people may face in attempting to improve their lot is well illustrated by the case of the I's. To them it seemed that the system had been designed in such a way that they were destined to remain poor. When one of their allowances was increased an equivalent amount was taken away from another allowance, and when they successfully applied for additional benefits they lost some of the discretionary payments to which they had been entitled. For example, when Family Allowance, paid to all families with children under 16 years, went up Mr I's invalidity benefit was reduced by an equivalent amount.

Mrs I: I thought it was a mistake in the books so I enquired and they said 'No, your family allowance went up.' 'Oh' I said. There was nothing . . . I couldn't argue with them, you know. If that goes up anymore he just loses it all the time, so we are no better off.

Int: Did they tell you why that had happened?

Mrs I: Well, it's automatic, it's just something they do, you know.

In this respect, families where the main wage earner is disabled are at a double disadvantage. Because they are dependent on state support they receive minimal financial resources and, unlike families where income is derived from work, increases in general benefits like family allowances have no effect on their total disposable income. Similarly, when Mr I was awarded an attendance allowance providing an additional £10 a week, he received a letter from the education authorities stating that their three children were no longer going to receive free school meals. Because they had not been given any reason why, they assumed that the two events were connected. Consequently, they were not sure that they would apply for further allowances in case this produced a similar outcome.

Mr I: I got a form through about a month ago about a mobility allowance I'm allowed but will it affect me rent rebate or anything like that 'cus they call that income, don't they? Well, I don't think that's fair, I don't think that's income, a mobility allowance, really that is to try and help me to get out and about, I don't see how it should come in with my income.

Int: Have you applied for that yet?

Mr I: No, I'm in two minds . . . I want to see what this rehab officer says when she comes here, explain to her and if she says 'Yeah, well, it'll come into your income,' I shan't apply for it 'cus that means I've got to pay more rent, it's going to affect my rebate, they'll probably turn round and say 'you can't have no more children's clothes allowance 'cus you're getting in so much over the top.' I've got a form in there to fill in but, as I say, we're just. . . . We don't know whether to send it off or not, we can't afford the money to go down anymore.

Given the difficulty that disabled people face in getting the welfare bureaucracy to respond to their self-perceived needs, they may give up the struggle to make ends meet and allow themselves to accumulate debts. Rising costs and static benefits may leave them with no other choice. At the second interview, Mr M said that his rent had risen by £5 a week while his invalidity benefit was not due to rise for a further five months.

Mr M: It's getting a major problem now just getting to make money meet everything you've got to do. It just isn't adding up, no way is that adding up. Even if I live the life of a monk it still won't add up so I don't always pay the rent, if something heavy comes up the rent won't be paid.

Int: Does that bother you?

Mr M: It used to but not now, I've got to the stage where I couldn't care two monkeys. I mean, you know, if I'm denied and I'm struggling to be honest and straightforward, no ruddy way. I might as well struggle on best I can. If I get in rent arrears I get in rent arrears now. I don't care, I take the attitude now if they refuse one way I take it another, my attitude is quite a simple one. I'm denied everything so I might as well start fiddling it my own best way. I used to worry about being 10 pence arrears in rent, that's gone now, that's going to be the last of the worries that.

Worrying about financial problems was one of the non-material consequences of attempting to live on an inadequate income and added an additional burden to be borne along with the other worries created by chronic illness. Prior to the second interview Mr M had been diagnosed as having a duodenal ulcer which he attributed to the stress caused by a lack of money. He said 'The problems you've got worrying about your bills plus your aches and pains, if those problems could be alleviated life would be a lot easier.' In fact the medication for his ulcer meant additional spending on medications, increasing somewhat the proportion of his income that had to be allocated to essential items. Mr F attributed much of the depression he suffered after giving up work to concern about his financial situation, and Mr H felt that this was having an effect on the chances of his recovery: 'This tends to worry me a lot and this doesn't help the treatment because I tend to lie and worry, you know, economically, and I don't really see how one can hope to get very well lying depressed.'

As well as coping with the worry of financial problems, disabled people and their families may also have to cope with the symbolic loss associated with poverty and dependency. As others have revealed, the stigma of receiving financial support from the state frequently means that entitlements are not claimed (Pinker and McLean 1974). Among this group Mrs A wished to avoid seeking help from Social Security following her retirement from work because, 'I was born in a very independent family and I'm not very keen on that.' Similarly, she had purchased whatever aids she needed because 'it didn't appeal to go cap in hand for charity'. Mrs R's daughter, who had never worked because of her mother's need for constant attention, refused to accept social security payments but accepted the invalid care allowance which she viewed as payment for her caring work. Even where people viewed allowances and discretionary payments as rights, stigma sometimes arose because the officials who administer the welfare bureaucracy dispensed moral condemnation along with services and benefits.

Perhaps the clearest illustration of the symbolic loss associated with poverty was that of the I's. Since Mr I became disabled and they both stopped work, Mrs I had struggled to maintain standards and present a respectable front to the outside world. She had no qualms about seeking the support of the State and had spent a lot of time trying to find out about, and trying to secure, those benefits to which she felt the family was entitled. However, she wished to conceal this dependency and loss of status from others and would not ask her family for assistance.

> *Mrs I:* I mean they feel sorry for us but there's nothing they can do, moneywise or anything. Well, I wouldn't ask. It's pride more than anything. I wouldn't ask 'em for nothing I wouldn't ask his family for anything.
> *Int:* Why?
> *Mrs I:* I wouldn't, I don't like to have people think I'm down. I mean I know I'm down, I mean, as long as my rent's paid and my children are fed, I don't care.

Such tactics may also be employed by children who seek to avoid loss of status by concealing the family's reduced circumstances and inability to pay for holidays and other desirable goods.

> *Mrs I:* They can't get used to it when all their friends say they're going away for a fortnight and these aren't going and they say 'My mum's going to take me out for days,' but they know damn well I'm not. You find the children are lying to their friends saying they are going out for days. They shouldn't do. They shouldn't have to say them things.

The need for children to preserve their status with their peers by acquiring what they defined as desirable goods and opportunities was recognized by Mr and Mrs I and imposed an additional burden on scarce resources. Consequently, the I's tried to make sure that their children were not disadvantaged or seen to be disadvantaged by others.

> *Mr I:* I mean, like my boy, my boy's 15 this year and my gel's 14, I mean, well, they want to be up to date with their friends now, you know, they come in and they want denims and cords and all that, and their shoes, God, their shoes are murder their shoes now and they've got to have shoes that go with their clothes and they work out at eight or nine pounds each.

The I's were only able to meet these needs by buying one item of clothing or footwear per week. In order to preserve equity within the family, the goods were not distributed until the full complement had been acquired.

> *Mrs I:* I bought my eldest daughter a pair of shoes last week, I

promised my little girl I'd buy her a pair this week and then my son next week. I can only do it that way, but I don't let the eldest wear hers until they've all got them 'cus, I mean, it wouldn't be fair. I said 'Once you've all got 'em, you can have 'em.'

Poverty may also call into question the adequacy of disabled parents and their spouses since it may prevent or make it more difficult for them to meet conventional criteria defining good parenthood. Parents are held responsible for providing for the material needs of their children, in particular, for making sure that they are adequately fed and adequately dressed. A failure to meet these needs may have implications for the moral identity and public image of the parents (Voysey 1975; Locker 1981). Consequently, though Mrs I could not really afford to buy meat every day, the money had to be found, ' 'cus there's no way my children are going out saying that don't have meals, I wouldn't do it'. Mrs I also refused to accept any decline in the quality of the clothing she bought for her children. In the effort to find sufficient money to maintain her standards, she went to the local Social Security Office and asked for an additional grant.

Mrs I: You know what they told me up there? They said 'there's plenty of jumble sales.' I said 'Is there? Well, you can go then 'cus I'm not giving my children jumble sale clothes.' Well, why should I put my kids in jumble sale clothes 'cus I don't know where they come from? She said 'Well, you just can't go in these big shops.' I said 'I'm not asking to go in big shops. I'm asking if you can help me to buy something reasonable.' I said 'Children like to have nice clothes and that's it.' That's when they turned round and told me to go to jumble sales. I mean, I know loads of people do but I just don't do it and that's it. I mean, you can't go and get shoes at jumble sales, you don't know what sort of feet people have had before my children had had them on their feet. My kids are my world and that's it.

For Mr and Mrs I, disability meant a lack of resources which in turn meant some difficulty in providing the things they believed children had a right to expect. As Mrs I said several times during the interviews, 'It's just not fair.' Later on, when talking about the possibility of her going back to work part-time, she said 'even if it's only for a couple of hours it'd be something to give my kids a holiday or something'.

6   Social contacts, social relationships, and family life

Some of the data presented in Chapters 2 to 5 has made passing reference to the impact of impairment and disability on social relationships and family life. This chapter attempts to examine this issue in more detail. I say attempts since the data on this topic is more limited than that which gave rise to the foregoing chapters. There are a number of reasons for this. One is that questions on these relatively sensitive topics were usually left until the end of the interview and were often curtailed because of the physical discomfort caused to the respondents by sitting in one position for two hours or more. Another was that questions asked tended to be vague and ill-defined, largely in an attempt to avoid causing distress or offence. It was often the case that problems in this area gave rise to more unhappiness than the practical problems of daily living, and this was particularly so when the respondents felt their disability had had an adverse effect on spouses, children, or others. Nevertheless, many of the respondents talked freely about their relationships with others, and in some cases no questioning was necessary; the descriptions emerged spontaneously during the course of the interview so that little probing was needed to stimulate further talk. As always, the concern was with the nature of the problems the respondents encountered and the resources and strategies they mobilized in the attempt to avoid or minimize them.

There is, of course, a large and growing literature dealing with disability and social relationships, emerging shortly after the Second World War and receiving added impetus from the studies of Goffman (1963) and Davis (1964). More recent work has concentrated on the family, documenting the burden imposed on others by the presence of a chronically sick or disabled person (Sainsbury and Grad de Alarcon 1974). The theme underlying this work is that disability impinges on others in a variety of ways and acts back on the disabled individual to reinforce and exacerbate their problems. While disability may disable the normal (Hilbourne 1973), rendering the rules of routine social interaction inapplicable, it is ultimately the disabled person who is the more severely disadvantaged. For the able-bodied, such problems occur in fleeting encounters and are unlikely to have any lasting impact on their identity or life chances. They are easily managed by withdrawing back into the world of the non-disabled. The disabled must, however, suffer these assaults on identity and may only withdraw into isolation or the narrow world of co-sufferers and consorts.

Legitimation

One problem common to many of the respondents, and there are some who would argue that it is common to all who lay claim to an acute or chronic illness (Parsons 1951; Haber and Smith 1971), is that of legitimation – having others accept the reality of their distress and the inevitability of the constraints imposed upon them. This requires others to define their complaints as valid indicators of their subjective experiences and their incapacity as disability created by a chronic condition and not wilful deviance (Haber and Smith 1971). This problem is not, as Parsons' original discussion might suggest, confined to the prediagnostic stage of the disease; it is never wholly resolved by the provision of a clinical label. Many of the respondents had been called upon to manage challenges to their experiences and actions long after they had been diagnosed as having rheumatoid arthritis and had been in specialist care. Doctors and other accredited gatekeepers may separate the disabled from the deviant during the diagnostic process but family, friends, colleagues, and strangers, even co-sufferers, while accepting the person's status as disabled, continue to monitor his or her performance in that role. The meaning of the diagnosis fluctuates, being negotiated and renegotiated over time.

Of course, the work done by the provision of the diagnosis depends largely upon the meaning of that diagnosis to others, influenced in turn by the public image of the disease and lay conceptions of its typical character and typical sufferers. Some may confuse rheumatoid arthritis with rheumatism and arthritis, the labels attached to relatively trivial joint pains common among the elderly and not so elderly. They then may wonder about individuals who claim to be severely disabled by these 'ordinary illnesses' and dismiss their claims to special status.

> *Mrs T:* I have had people literally say to me 'Erm, my dear girl, whatever's the matter? Whatever have you done to yourself? Have you had polio?' and I'd say 'No, rheumatoid arthritis.' 'Oh rheumatism,' and lose interest immediately. I've never understood it, it used to amuse me in fact because while I don't think rheumatoid arthritis is as serious as polio it does have very bad crippling effects but it was this complete loss of interest and I remember one lady said 'Oh yes, my grandfather used to get that in his shoulder.'

Revealing a diagnosis to others may fail to secure legitimation for a given incapacity simply because the person concerned is believed by others to fall outside the category of individuals who get the disease. For example, arthritic complaints are usually thought to be diseases of the elderly; Mrs D's response to being told she had rheumatoid arthritis at the age of 14 was one of, 'Gawd, that's an old woman's complaint, I can't have that.' Consequently, younger people may simply not be believed. Mrs W had often encountered people who said, 'Are you sure you've got arthritis?', and Mr K, whose wife had multiple sclerosis as well as arthritis, had also experienced this problem.

> *Mr K:* I've had one or two people try to be funny. I had a bloke in the road just before we moved here and he said to me, 'Your wife's drunk,' and I said 'Say that again and I'll break your bloody neck. She's got MS.' 'I've heard that before' he said. You, know a lot of people turn round and say 'No woman of her age, she couldn't possibly have MS.'

The extent to which others are prepared to confer legitimacy upon the suffering and incapacity of those with a chronic disorder is influenced by two factors, the character of the relationship between them and the character of the disorder responsible for the person's limited activity. As Wiener (1975) has suggested, other people often have stakes in the arthritic person remaining active so may not be prepared to accept the legitimacy of his or her complaints. Questioning the validity of their experiences and actions may involve less disruption to their own lives and avoids the necessity of giving support (Locker 1981). The problem is exacerbated in an illness like rheumatoid arthritis because the main symptom, pain, is an intangible phenomenon not directly available to others. In the early stages, it is often not accompanied by any signs which would help to verify the sufferer's complaints. Moreover, while individuals may be subject to severe and continuous pain, they are often unable to convey the experience to others in the form of a description; people with rheumatoid arthritis find it difficult to say exactly where and how much it hurts and may even find it difficult to locate the pain exactly (Bury 1976). In short, they find it difficult to make others understand their pain. This can often result in as much distress as the physical discomfort itself.

> *Mr F:* While it was developing, well, it could really unbalance you. It is, as I say, you can't explain the pain, so nobody, if you've never had it. . . . It's not like a toothache, you know. If you've got a toothache then people can probably sympathize with you and know what it's like but with this rheumatoid arthritis pain, I dunno. The only experience I can liken it to was, you know, in the army when you used to have to run around with a rifle over your head and every bone in your body. aches, that is the only way I could explain it. But you try to explain it to

your wife and kids, you know. There was no physical illness there that they could see and they couldn't understand that you were in pain all the time, that you wanted to be left alone. That was the worst part.

The difficulty of having others understand and accept the extent of the pain often allowed the person's associates to challenge the legitimacy of the experience and the limitations to which it gave rise.

Mrs R: I used to pray and wish with all my heart that there was some kind of machine that would measure pain because I thought no one in the world can understand the pain of rheumatoid arthritis, you know. Often I used to say if only someone would come along with a machine to measure pain 'cus you can't get people to understand. I mean, my sister, I know she didn't believe me for the simple reason that I'd have pain in the morning and as soon as it had gone I'd be off, I was full of life, I loved life. She used to say to me 'You can't be in pain all the time, no one's in pain all the time.'

Miss L: I felt nobody understood me, I know it sounds awful but I thought you don't know how painful it can be when I'd try to lift something up and they'd say 'Surely, you can do that?' and I thought 'You don't know what it's like.' But, of course, they don't know and how can they know.

The only source of understanding seems to come from co-sufferers or others with similarly painful conditions who have had similar experiences. Mrs J's brother also had rheumatoid arthritis and was her main source of support; Miss L had a friend with a painful, disabling condition of the spine, 'She understands completely and absolutely'; and the sister who figured in the account given by Mrs R had recently been diagnosed as having arthritis, 'She rings me up now crying, sometimes she'll say "I'm never out of pain." Well, I can't be hard because I know the pain.'

Another characteristic of rheumatoid arthritis which makes for difficulty in securing legitimacy is the day-to-day variation in levels of pain and activity. Taking advantage of a good day to get out and about may make the inactivity of a bad day difficult to justify. Similarly, the efforts of people with arthritis to master pain and keep going may lead others to believe that, when temporarily unable to do so, they are lying or exaggerating the extent of their pain. As Wiener's respondents discovered, success at concealing their illness and striving to maintain normal levels of activity was a mixed blessing; normalization minimized the impact of the illness on their lives but gave rise to problems when the façade could not be sustained in the face of an acute flare-up. Part of Mrs R's difficulty arose because she would maximize activity whenever levels of pain would allow, and Mr M felt that his doctors did not believe his complaints because some days he was relatively mobile.

Int: Did they say anything about your back?

Mr M: No. I don't think they believed me, quite honestly, or at least I got that impression.

Int: What made you think that?

Mr M: Because although I'm in pain I can bend reasonably, er, I can bend. Although it hurts to bend I can bend a little bit and I felt that the attitude is 'Oh, if he can bend he can't be as bad as all that.' There is a certain amount of stiffness there but like anything else good days and bad days and if you go there on what you might call a reasonably good day where you can bend I don't think they believe you.

With time, the presence and seriousness of rheumatoid arthritis may become visible either through obvious deformity in hands or limbs or the necessity to use an aid such as a stick or a wheelchair. Mrs T considered herself fortunate that the gravity of her situation had rarely been challenged but ascribed that to the fact that her illness was readily apparent: 'It's only a fool who's going to look at these hands and think they got like that free of cost.' By contrast, Mrs G was continually exasperated by the tendency of others to underestimate her problems, minimize the extent of her pain, and fail to provide the help she needed. Despite being severely disabled, there was little sign of this until it became necessary to use a wheelchair. At one time she had been particularly hurt by a nurse's casual remark.

Mrs G: I dare say she wasn't thinking because there again you see it doesn't show that I can't see, you see it doesn't show that I can't feel and people do understand, say, an amputation better than a pair of legs that don't work because it doesn't show. These legs don't look sick, my hands don't look sick, my eyes don't look sick, right? I don't look sick. Crazily, once you're in a chair, things they can see, they can sympathize with once you're in a chair, not that I want to be in one. Now they're beginning to understand this lady's sick so the caring gets bigger, you know what I mean, er. . . . All the time you can hop around and, as my son said when he came here last time, they see me sitting here like this, he went away and his last words were 'You're all right now', you see, because it doesn't show.

The problem of legitimation is not confined to the reality or severity of symptoms but extends to the behavioural responses to those symptoms. Even though others may accept that a person is chronically sick and disabled, the extent and origins of his or her limitations may still be questioned. They may be seen to be making too much of their illness and exaggerating the disability it produces. Paradoxically, such criticism could be a source of distress or a source of help; it was distressing when the person was unable to rise above his or her pain and do more but helpful when it prevented the individual from succumbing to the disorder. At the second interview Mrs T agonized about the burden placed on her husband now that she was virtually bedbound and was grateful for the generosity of his response.

> *Mrs T:* It does put a tremendous burden on his shoulders because what it does mean is he's carrying both of us. He comes home of a night and I've been up about a quarter of an hour or sometimes I just stay in bed and there's never any difference, he doesn't get irritable with me, he never makes the slightest suggestion either by word or even by look that I could do a little better if I tried and that perhaps I ought to try and make more effort, nothing like that, which is an absolute godsend because if he did I just don't know how I'd live with it because when you're making the greatest effort that you can anyway and your greatest effort means that you're lying in bed smiling weakly I think if someone were to say 'I think you really ought to pull your socks up a bit' I don't know how I'd manage.

On the other hand Mrs X had been helped by such criticism from family and friends and their refusal to allow her to slip into a dependent role. She had spent five years confined to a wheelchair but was now able to walk around outside without help. Friends had worked hard to prevent her from becoming housebound, saying 'pull yourself together' and forcing her to go out despite her pain, and her daughters had not allowed her to exaggerate her need for help but maximized her capacity for independent living. As Mrs X said, 'I have been inclined to swing it on the poor devils at times but they've been very firm, they've said "No, mum, you do it yourself, we're not going to do it. Make the effort, you do it." ' The ease with which encouragement and criticism can become confused readily creates the conditions for the growth of tension and conflict. Although in this case the outcome was positive, it had only been attained at the cost, albeit temporary, of a deterioration in family relationships. As Mrs X continued, 'I love my family dearly, but at times I don't like them very much.'

Coping by withdrawal

For many of the respondents coping with pain often meant coping alone. Partly because others could not understand their pain and partly because the effort of managing pain consumed already depleted reserves of energy, leaving little to be invested in routine interaction, most withdrew from the company of others and preferred to be alone. This withdrawal took a number of forms and was designed to manage a number of problems. Some resolved the problem of legitimating the reality of their pain by ceasing to reveal to others the extent of their suffering. Mrs R and

Mr S chose to head off challenges to the validity of their complaints by staying silent, saying 'I just kept it to myself' and 'I don't moan with the pain. They know I've got it but I don't let them know I've got it. I just do what I always do and that's it.' Some also withdrew into themselves when they were unable to participate in interaction but found it difficult to withdraw physically. At work Miss L sometimes went quiet: 'People will say "What's wrong with you?" It's just that you don't feel like laughing and joking.' Many, however, would withdraw physically, separating themselves from family and friends until the pain had begun to subside. There were a number of reasons for this. One was the difficulty of coping with pain and engaging in social intercourse at the same time, another that the effort of maintaining a normal front while in the company of others was just too great and another that they often did not bother to wash or dress when in pain and had no wish to be seen in that state by anyone other than close family.

> *Mrs T:* When I'm in pain I don't want to see anyone because it means I have to make an effort to talk to them, obviously if someone comes to see you you can't say 'Look, I'm feeling under the weather today and I don't want to talk to you,' and have them sit in a chair and read a paper. You can't do that and when I have got a lot of pain it takes so much of my energy to talk to people and I prefer not to. In any case when I'm feeling like that I often don't bother to get dressed I certainly don't make my face up and, well, naturally I'm the same as anybody else when I'm going to see somebody even though I might be under the weather I like to look as reasonable as I can so I'm not overstruck on seeing people. It's different with my husband, I always feel a little bit better when he's here, but then, of course I don't have to make so much effort with him, I don't have to put on a front.

Some of the respondents withdrew because they found it difficult to be civil to family and friends when in severe pain and some because the anxiety of others to help was a major source of irritation. In both cases keeping out of the way helped to minimize overt conflict.

> *Mrs J:* When I'm a bit down I don't want to talk to nobody and I don't want nobody to talk to me. I just want to be left completely alone to stew in my own misery, I just want to be left. I can't be bothered to get washed, dressed, or anything else, I slum it. I did Saturday, I was proper miserable. I just felt rotten and I was rotten, I didn't want to be bothered with anybody's questions. I don't do it deliberately but I can't be civil to anybody, I snap and bite, I'm really a pig. I just wish they'd leave me alone so I'm very curt.

> *Mr F:* It was the constant questioning all the time that used to get on my nerves. Where are you paining? How does it feel? You don't look

too good. You know, a couple of times they had me buried and that really used to get me going so if someone used to walk in I'd get up and walk out.

Int: Were you like that with the kids or your wife as well?

Mr F: Oh, my wife as well, or even when anybody, friends, came in I used to get up and walk out.

Of course, withdrawing from social interaction in order to cope with pain was not entirely without costs. Mr F said he had lost a number of friends because he was unable to tolerate their presence on his off days and others told of similar breaches in social relations. A few were fortunate in that family and friends assisted in their strategy of withdrawing and understood sufficiently to curtail visits or abandon outings as and when necessary. Mrs T had many friends of long standing who never called on the off chance but telephoned first or waited to be invited. With acquaintances who were not party to this arrangement she would not answer the door, pretending to be out rather than having to turn people away. At the second interview she said that the flat upstairs was occupied by three young men who were so anxious to assist that they always rushed to open the front door if they heard her bell being rung. Consequently, she was having to entertain unwanted visitors yet was at a loss as to how she might explain to the new tenants that she would prefer not to have their help. She was looking forward to moving to a flat with its own front door so she could regain control over her territory and maintain her strategy intact.

Stigma and identity spread

Despite Goffman's initial statement (Goffman 1963) and subsequent empirical elaborations, stigma remains difficult to define. At its simplest level it refers to the attribution of inferiority and unacceptability by others to someone 'marked' in some way. In the case of the chronically ill this marking may be obvious deformity, ungainly or unco-ordinated movements, or the necessity to use the paraphernalia of disability such as sticks, crutches, or wheelchairs. The likelihood that a chronically ill person will be stigmatized by others is, in part, a function of the specific disease, its manifestations, and its effects. As Blaxter has suggested, some may be stigmatized more by the consequences of a disorder, for example unemployment and poverty, than by the disorder itself. A number of factors are likely to be involved in the development of stigma; prominent among them are the social image of the particular disease and its visibility. Some diseases are 'clean' and some polluting and unwholesome (Shearer 1981), some are readily apparent because of their effects on the body, and some are not visible to others. Persons with diseases such as heart conditions may not be stigmatized because their problem is common, 'clean', largely invisible, and unlikely to intrude on social interaction. People with leprosy or multiple sclerosis may find themselves in quite a different situation. The issue of visibility is a crucial one. Those with disorders which do not have external manifestations can head off stigma by information control, though they may have to cope with the fear of being found out. Those with a visible impairment have little to gain by information control but must use alternative strategies for managing strained interaction when it occurs (Davis 1964). Rheumatoid arthritis is not visible during its early stages and only becomes noticeable when joint or limb deformity develops or it becomes necessary to use sticks and the like. Even in its later stages the disease may be easy to conceal; Mrs J said 'If I was to put a coat on and gloves on nobody would now there was anything wrong with me.' At times this can be a mixed blessing. On the one hand it means that information control can be used to conceal the presence of the disorder, at least until it becomes apparent by an inability to perform routine daily tasks. On the other hand it may mean that falling in public or struggling to get on a bus are readily misinterpreted. Mrs I had often had to explain to reluctant taxi drivers that her husband needed to be helped into the cab because he had arthritis, not because he was drunk. Mr P's inability to grip small objects had also been misinterpreted on occasions.

> *Mr P:* When I went to the doctor's one time the receptionist gave me the prescription. Well, she give it to me and it just went through me hand onto the floor and she went straight in and reported me to the doctor and said 'He threw it on the floor.'

Perhaps because rheumatoid arthritis can be concealed by most sufferers most of the time, the respondents who presented accounts of stigmatizing encounters tended to be those who used wheelchairs or those who had visible physical deformity. For them, their impairment and disability often became the central focus of interaction with the non-disabled. It is worth remembering, however, that not all encounters between disabled people and others are stigmatizing, even when the focus is on their disability. Far from it. Mrs O, for example, told of encounters which had had a positive impact on her sense of worth.

> *Mrs O:* I mean, I was in Sainsbury's this morning and a gentleman tapped me on the shoulder, I'd never seen him before, he said 'I think you're wonderful.' 'Oh,' I said 'thank you very much.' 'Yes, I do' he said 'I've watched you, I think it's marvellous how you get around and do your shopping and drive that little car, 'cus' he said 'my wife's got arthritis and can't get out.' It happens a lot to me, you know, people telling me how good I am, complete strangers. I think it's lovely. I think, well, perhaps, you know, I am good.

Despite positive encounters of this kind, a few of the respondents were sensitive about their appearance because it singled them out from the crowd, drew unwanted attention, or caused others to treat them in undesirable ways. Miss L said 'You don't want to go hobbling down the road like an old lady, you feel people are looking at you' and even Mrs O said 'I don't like going anywhere where I've got to walk in front of people. I like to sit in a corner.' Mr P felt that his physical deformity was an impediment to making contacts with others and felt ostracized by some of the people at his day centre: 'They look at you, they look at your bent fingers and bent hands, there's other people there with arthritis who'll talk to you but the others don't want to know.' Of course, chronically sick people may be the recipients of special attention even when their condition is not visible to others simply because their associates are aware of their problem and take it into account. This special consideration can be very helpful but at times can also be subtly degrading. For example, Mr I was no longer just one of a group of mates who used the same pub.

> *Mr I:* They'll give me a stool now rather than keep it for themselves, one of me mates who knows me, knows what I'm like, will get off their stool which they wouldn't have done before. Well, I find that . . . well, say it's in my mind, but I know they don't take a drink off me now. At one time they would. They send me one over and I go to send one and, 'Oh no, don't you dare,' like.

The kind of encounters this group of people found to be stigmatizing were those which resulted in what can be called identity spread (Strauss 1975). Here one characteristic of the person is taken to characterize the person as a whole. Consequently, the individual stops being a person or a person with a disability who may need special consideration some of the time and becomes a disabled person, identified solely by his or her medical problem and the limitations it imposes. Their disability becomes the pivot around which interaction with others revolves. Opening remarks by these others frequently take the form of enquiries about the disorder and subsequent talk may consist of this topic alone and exclude all others. Several of the respondents found this very irritating and tried to prevent their medical problems overriding all other concerns by avoiding them in conversation with others. In this way they tried to avoid having their disabled status constantly reaffirmed in routine encounters.

Another form of identity spread that may emerge during social encounters is something best described as the assumption of general incompetence. The difficulties a disabled person has with some of the activities of everyday living are generalized by the non-disabled to *all* activities, whether physical or cognitive. The people in wheelchairs in particular seemed to find that obvious signs of physical disability were often taken to mean an associated mental disability as well. This took one of two forms; the crude form can be illustrated by the following accounts.

Mrs W: There were a group of us, some had MS and some had other things and we were sitting next to these people and they offered to buy ice cream and I said 'No thank you' and they said 'Excuse me asking but which home are you from?' I said 'My own.' She gives a look and I say 'And so are they.' And as I turned away I heard her say 'I thought they were all from some mental institution.' I said 'My God, that's all we need' and she heard it and was really annoyed. But I didn't enlighten her, I just said 'my own home' and left it at that.

A more subtle form of this assumption of incompetence is the 'Does he take sugar?' syndrome in which it is assumed that disabled people are incapable of responding to questions about their capacities and needs. A number of respondents found it very annoying when people would bypass them in conversation.

Mrs T: I have got a little bit irritable when people have asked my mother or my husband if I'm sitting comfortably. My mother just used to look across at me and wait for me to answer but Frank will say 'Why don't you ask her?' You know, 'Is Mary warm enough? Is she in a draught?' That's why we love the title of that radio programme, *Does he take sugar?* We thought that was brilliant. No one has ever asked Frank if I take sugar but on numerous occasions they've said to him 'Is it all right if Mary has some gin?' It's extraordinary that people think that because you can't use your legs properly in someway it's affected your understanding so you don't know if you're in a draught or your chair's comfortable or if you're too near the fire.

Such is the frequency with which these things happen that some of the respondents had misinterpreted the comments of others, seeing them as instances of identity spread or the assumption of incompetence when they were not. Even more difficult interactional situations may then arise. At one social function Mrs W got so tired of people approaching her to ask if she had multiple sclerosis that she gave up telling them about arthritis and thought she would say nothing.

Mrs W: Then this chap came up and said 'How long have you had MS?' 'Oh, years' I said. 'Have you?' he said. 'Oh yes, years,' I said. So he says 'That's funny, it took my sister differently, she can hardly speak and she wets herself.' 'O God,' I thought 'what have I done now?' I couldn't tell him I didn't have it.

Mrs R had also found herself in situations where she had misunderstood a question or comment reading it as a derogatory remark when it was not.

Mrs R: I had to go round to the solicitor to have an affadavit sworn and he came out to the car and said 'Can you write?' 'O God, we're not going to start all of *that* over again.' And then he went back and Carol went in to pay him and he said 'Hasn't she got arthritis badly? Isn't that a terrible complaint?' So you see it can be misconstrued.

These interactional difficulties were easier to handle in the company of a close associate such as a spouse or child. Mrs R and her daughter had a routine whereby they would force others into treating Mrs R as a person rather than an incompetent, and Mrs T's husband was 'quite wicked' in those situations and never failed to poke fun at people who were offensive through ignorance. The effects of the encounters were neutralized by turning them into stories illustrating the stupidity of normals; as Mrs R said 'We've often had a laugh over that.' Nevertheless, such encounters do have an impact, and at times Mrs R would prefer not to be seen in her chair.

Mrs R: Really it's pride, it is pride. You see, when I'm sitting in the car I feel normal, and if people do come to speak to me they don't speak to me as if I'm. . . I've noticed when I go out in my car, erm, there's one or two neighbours that speak to us and they speak to you just normally, they don't treat me as though I'm an invalid at all.

Her house was constructed in a way that allowed her to go unobserved from the house to the garage so that by the time she came within view she was in the driving seat, in control of her car, and able to pass as normal.

Isolation and confinement

The pattern of social contacts enjoyed by this group of respondents varied from individual to individual and was influenced by a number of factors such as household composition, marital status, the extent of available social networks, and degrees of disability. On the one hand, some of the people managed to get out of the house once a day unless forced to stay indoors by bad weather or an acute flare-up, and on the other, people like Mrs G and Mrs T rarely went out at all. At the first interview, Mrs T had been out no more than four times in the previous seven months, and by the time of the second interview she had left the house twice in six months, and one of those was a visit to her general practitioner. Some of the individuals were isolated and lonely, and some were confined within their homes. The two did not always go together so that those most confined were not necessarily isolated or lonely and vice versa. As might be expected it was the single and widowed with few family contacts who were the loneliest people within the group even though they were not necessarily stranded in their homes. In fact, these people tended to go out rather more than some of those who lived with family. The reason for this was that loneliness had driven them to take advantage of luncheon clubs, day centres for the disabled, and meetings of voluntary organizations in order to break the monotony and isolation of their lives. Most used these facilities twice a week or more and would have used them more often if transport had been available. Though not ideal as sources of recreational activity, these organizations did provide the opportunity to get out of the house and enjoy the company of others. At other times, however, they did have to put up with loneliness and isolation, as did many who lived with family but spent the majority of weekdays alone. For example, Mrs V looked forward to the two days she was taken by ambulance to a local luncheon club but did not go out the rest of the week: 'It's not much thrill really sitting here hour after hour on your own.' Weekends seemed long and empty and Sundays were days when isolation became almost complete.

> *Mrs V:* I loathe Sundays 'cus the street's quiet and you don't see the traffic and the people backwards and forwards and I don't see anybody. Sunday's always very miserable.

Mrs N was married, lived with her husband, and had two daughters who often came to visit but still found the days were lonely: 'It's just sitting here all day long looking at the houses over the road. There's nobody in and it's so boring and sometimes there's all evening to face as well.' Mrs W was also married and heavily involved in activities for the disabled and local political life, sometimes having to attend three or more meetings a week, yet still felt the effects of being confined. She only went out when a car was available to collect her and dearly wished that she could get out on her own.

> *Mrs W:* I'd like to be able to get out, I don't like being caged in, I don't like being shut in here. Now as the weather gets warmer and brighter I'll get sadder. It's terrible really. They all say 'Look at it,' and I think 'God, I'm stuck in here' and then I begin to think 'What a life, I'm stuck here.' And it's worse in the summer. When my husband's home he takes me out weekends and that's something but then I'm back in on Mondays and I often say to him, 'Can't you have the day off work and we'll go out?' and he says 'You can't do that these days. You lose too much money.' So I'm back where I started and that makes me miserable. And if anybody says the sun shining makes you happy it doesn't me, it makes me the reverse. If it's miserable and cold and raining I feel better 'cus I wouldn't want to go out in that so that's all right. I get more lonely in the summer when I see all the people out and about 'cus you think 'If only I could go out.'

The reasons for the development of isolation are many and complex but include the disposition of the individual, the availability of resources, the robustness of their social networks, and the problems of opportunity and access. Withdrawal as a mechanism for coping with pain is one source of social isolation within the family. Another form of withdrawal is that which leads to the separation of the individual from the wider world of the 'normal'. This is largely a response to embarrassment and stigma (Cunningham 1977). Recreational activities may be avoided and social contacts reduced because they highlight the disability and disadvantage of the person concerned. Mr F had given up going to his usual pubs and clubs because of this.

> *Mr F:* You go out, especially with a stick or a couple of sticks, and people, they're looking at you and I feel embarrassed about it and I just don't feel like going where there are people, possibly this is the reason I don't go to the pub because I'll usually drink a pint but I can't pick up a pint glass it's impossible without both of my hands, I go up like that, they think you're a wino or something. I get the needle sometimes . . . I know they don't mean any harm by it but I could do without it. I used to go to this club, but I don't like going down now. They're all dancing and you're hopping about with a stick, you can't lift a pint, you feel a bit out of place.

Nowadays, going out meant sitting just outside the front door reading a newspaper in the sunshine or, in winter, taking the car up to the local park and watching people play football.

Not all deliberately avoided social contacts but became isolated for one or more other reasons. During periods of severe pain, going out would be reduced because it was impossible to summon the energy needed to get ready and get out. At other times the effort involved also proved to be too much.

> *Mrs T:* I went out to dinner with some friends in April and I haven't been out since. I can't make the effort. When I'm sitting here in my nightie my husband says 'Would you like to go for a drive around?' and I think to myself, 'O God, I've got to get washed and dressed and make my face up' and it seems so much to do, so much effort that I'll say 'Let's see what it's like tomorrow' and he doesn't push it. I just don't think about going out now, it doesn't cross my mind except my husband will persevere, he will give me the option to keep it in my mind and remind me 'cus God knows when was the last time I said 'I'd like to go out.' But it is brought about mostly by lack of energy.

Mrs R often avoided going out because it sometimes involved a great deal of effort for her daughter. Because she felt her daughter already had enough to do in providing care and managing the house, she was unwilling to burden her further by making additional demands on her time and energy. The necessity of being helped to go out also acted as a constraint on the social activities of many other respondents. The more severely disabled needed help simply to get out of the house, the less severely disabled needed help if they were to go further than the length of the street. Some required the help of other people, some required the use of a car, and some required both. If these resources were not available then the individual concerned had to stay home. Prior to one interview Mr M had been on a trip to the coast, 'but only because they collected me at the door', whereas Mrs G was unable to take advantage of a similar trip organized by the residents of the block of flats in which she lived because of a lack of help.

> *Mrs G:* You see, if I go out it's literally door to door, somebody picks me up and lifts me in. Next Tuesday there's an outing from here to Brighton but I daren't go because it means getting on a coach right. There's steps about a foot high and there's nobody to lift me in and nobody to lift me out and even if I'm allowed to take the chair, and there are a couple of flies in the ointment who say 'No chairs', supposing I could take the chair, I'd still need to be lifted in 'cus there are seven or eight steps up to the hotel where we have lunch. Then there's nobody to push me from there to the convenience, or whatever, so I've decided not to go which is rather sad as it only happens once a year.

Mr and Mrs H had no living relatives and no car and, unlike many of the disabled people living in the same block, were confined to the block and its immediate environment.

> *Mrs H:* You see, a lot of people here have got cars and a couple of men to heave them in and out. A lot more drive their own cars because they've got the hands and arms and can heave themselves in and out. But I'm stuck because I've got no hands, arms, feet, or anything. You see, they have to heave me about like a sack of potatoes. Well, a woman can't do this on her own, my wife can't, even if we'd got a car, she couldn't get me in and out of the thing in any case. You see it needs a couple of strong lads like yourself to put me in and take me out again. So one just has to live as we live, a very restricted life. If we had relatives it would make all the difference.

Even where help is available it might be erratic or not available when most needed. The person on the receiving end has little choice but to take the help as and when it comes and is often unable to exercise any degree of control; where they are dependent on others they have little option but to fit in with someone else's plans. The only time Mr I got out during the week was on a Wednesday evening when friends arrived with a car to take him round the corner to the pub. Mrs I said 'It's annoying to think he can't even manage from here round the corner' because that meant they did not go out if their friends chose to go elsewhere. The week prior to the interview their friends did not arrive so they stayed home, and they were uncertain what was to happen this week: 'They might be down tomorrow, we'll just have to see if they turn up or not.' Mr I was also unable to travel the short distance to see his family, and the only time he saw them was if they decided to visit him.

Nearly all of the respondents were conscious of the need to get out of the house, maintain their social contacts, inject some variety into their daily lives, and prevent their homes from becoming the limits of their world. Even Mrs T, who no longer thought of going out, was very worried by this and somewhat concerned lest it become a way of life from which she would never escape. She castigated herself saying 'I should make the effort, you shouldn't allow four walls to become a prison which is what I've already done.' Consequently, some engaged in activities, not because they valued the activity *per se*, but because they helped promote these other more important ends. Mr F sometimes took the opportunity of spending the day at his former place of work although he had given up trying to be of any help. He spent most of the time there sitting in a corner chatting to whoever happened to be around: 'Well, it's a day out. It's just to get out of the house mostly.' Similarly, Mrs V continued to go to meetings of the local branch of the Arthritis Association despite the fact that it involved a lot in the way of worry and inconvenience:

Mrs V: It's somewhere to go. I get fed up at times but it's still somewhere to go when you can't get out.
Int: Why do you get fed up?
Mrs V: It's not enough for one thing, it's not long enough. The anxiety of waiting for the ambulance and that, I get worked up in such a state. Sometimes they don't get here until half past seven so we don't get there till nearly eight o'clock and the thing is over at nine. So you get yourself really worked up and half the time it's not really worth it, but it's still somewhere to go and they are kind so I shall continue to go as long as the ambulance takes me.

Despite their efforts to get out and retain some sort of social life, the problems and barriers they had to face caused a dramatic decline in the frequency and quality of the respondents' social and recreational lives. That decline was also experienced by spouses who were equally disadvantaged in becoming isolated and confined. For example, Mr I was very active socially until the onset of disability.

Mr I: I used to see my family regular, never missed, every week. I used to go round Sunday with my brothers take my dad out for a drink Sunday lunchtime. But now I only see them when they come down to me now. I used to be out regular. I used to go to the pub over the road. I was always over there before I had this. I was always active. I was secretary of the darts club over there and everything, go to meetings twice a week, down Battersea Town Hall watching the matches and that. That's all stopped, I can't even get down there. I was very active at one time.

The change in the character of Mr I's social life and relations with others was highlighted by his response to a question concerning his current contacts with his old associates. When asked if he still saw his friends he said 'Oh yes . . . when was it? Sunday . . . going past there . . . we had the window open and they all yelled like, a few of them I used to know from across the way.' Mr I was waiting to move house and hoped he would be placed near to relatives because he thought this would increase his social contacts and lessen his isolation: 'If we lived just around the corner we'd see more of them.'

Dependency and help

One of the most significant transformations that may occur in the relationship between a disabled person and others is the development of dependence and the necessity to rely on help. The pain of being, or the fear of becoming, dependent were voiced by many of the respondents, particularly the more disabled who had to have help from spouses or children with personal care and other practicalities of daily life. Even those who were relatively independent and still able to do much in the way of caring for themselves and the household in which they lived still disliked having to ask for help. Mrs N, who was one of the least disabled of the respondents, only needed help with housework but found it 'awful having to depend on others to do things'. The few currently able to manage largely by themselves were fearful of a future which seemed to offer the prospect of increasing helplessness and dependency, and this fear was particularly acute among those who had personal experience of caring for people with a severe disability. Miss L had spent a number of years caring for her bed-ridden mother and was fully aware of the impact this could have on both: 'So I worry about becoming incapacitated and someone having to wait on me. Mother was exhausting and I don't want to be a burden, that does frighten me.'

Being dependent upon others gives rise to a number of problems, practical, symbolic, and psychological. Perhaps the most immediate problem is that even simple tasks can only be completed when someone is available and able to find the time to help. Dependency often means that it is necessary to wait until much needed help can be fitted into someone else's timetable, and until then the job simply remains undone. Not only does this give rise to the frustration of always having to wait, but it also heightens the sense of frustration at being trapped in a body no longer able to perform on cue. Tension and conflict may be generated between the person giving and the person receiving help, particularly where the two do not share the same methods of doing things or perform at the same pace. While strangers or distant associates may remain unaware of this, family members are often told. Mrs R, in talking about friction between herself and her daughter, said 'Carol's very slow, that's her nature, and I'm afraid I'm the opposite.' Of course, conflict that arises because help is not available at the exact moment it is needed or not given in exactly the right way may make the recipients appear and feel too demanding (Shearer 1981) so that they remain silent until the build up of tension results in an outburst they often regret. This transformation in social relationships is perhaps most acutely felt by those who had once been proud of their independence and been givers rather than receivers. For them, feelings of being a burden and feeling useless were particularly hard to bear.

Mrs R: When you've been independent all your life it's very hard you see, I find it very hard having to ask Carol to do everything. This is the hardest part of my life with her but I couldn't do without her.

Another problem the long-term sick and dependent may have to come to terms with is being a burden on someone else and seriously affecting the quality of his or her life. This is the case even where help is given willingly and without complaint. There were three instances among the group of respondents in this study where a spouse or child had taken on a full-time caring role. Mr H's wife was in constant attendance and rarely left him, Mr K had given up work to care for Mrs K, and Mrs R's daughter had left school when only 15 and for the past nine years had been increasingly responsible for providing for the needs of her mother and their household. Of the three, Mrs R was perhaps the most distressed by the effects of her need for constant care. Her case is worth examining in some detail since shortly after the second interview her daughter and son-in-law left and she was taken, albeit temporarily, into residential care. In fact, Mrs R's opening comments at the first interview addressed this very topic:

Mrs R: I couldn't do without my daughter and this is a big worry because, you know, you get to my age and you feel rather a burden because you've got a couple of youngsters here, they only got married last year. But she's so good and I'm very dependent on her which perhaps I shouldn't be quite so much but I couldn't manage without her, I'd be in a home without her there's no question of that.

Throughout the two interviews she returned to the same issue a number of times and elaborated further at a third interview she requested following her return home from residential care. The following quotes are taken from the initial interviews.

Mrs R: Carol does everything you see, and I honestly get to the stage where I think to myself 'I'll go into a home,' because, you know, why should I . . . ? I mean she's a very competent typist, her husband is very very clever, there's nothing he can't do and he wants to set up on his own. Well, Carol should be helping him but, erm, you know, this burden feeling this feeling of burden it's a terrible feeling.
Int: Even you feel that way?
Mrs R: Oh terrible at times. I've lay in bed and visualized packing a case and getting myself off and I've thought of doing it because why should I monopolize their lives, you know? How can you put it. . . ? It's a guilt complex the whole time. It's a selfish feeling. You think 'Well, I've had my life, why shouldn't they have theirs?' I don't think it's fair that she should have to give up all she's given up to look after me. I'm very grateful and she knows that. We're very close but now and again I do get a bit awkward and I get to the stage where, 'I don't want you to do that for me.' You know, it's pride coming out. But I've got a very good daughter and a very good son-in-law and if he begrudged the time she spent with me that would be terrible. In fact, if Carol and I quarrel and I get one of my moods and say 'I don't want you to do that,' which is natural, you get pride, he'll do it for me.

Not only was Mrs R concerned that her daughter's life chances had been adversely affected by her adoption of a caring role, she was also very concerned that Carol rarely went out. This arose partly because she felt it abnormal for a young woman to be confined with her mother and also because it reflected on her own public character.

Mrs R: You see, Carol won't go out much and the neighbours think it's through me that she doesn't go out but I've tried . . . one neighbour over the road rang me up and said 'Would Carol like to go to a show?' Well, she didn't want to go and instead of her getting on the phone and saying 'I don't want to go' I had to ring up and I said 'Carol is married.' And they said 'We know, but she doesn't go out much.' You see the only outing she gets is when we go round the shops or something like that. But she doesn't go out enough I don't think. You know, when they go out I love it but they're no sooner gone than they're back, it's not as if they stayed out for a long time. This is a big problem that I'd like to think there's some solution to but you can't force people out, can you? Sometimes I get cross, I get into a temper sometimes, I say 'Why don't you go out? Leave me alone! Get off out!' She says 'I don't want to go out.' So there's nothing you can do. At the same time it isn't normal for a young girl of 24 to be stuck in all the time with me. I don't know how that will solve itself.

Despite the lack of evidence to suggest that Carol wanted to go out more, her unwillingness to leave the house and Mrs R's failure to force her to live more of an independent existence seemed to increase Mrs R's sense of being a burden. She also seemed to believe that outsiders defined the situation in that way too; during the third interview she looked back at the breakdown in their relationship and said 'I felt that people were saying "This isn't right for a young girl." '

The relationship between helper and helped is one fraught with difficulty even when it is parent and child or spouse and spouse who occupy the roles. It is not only difficult in itself but made even more difficult by the fact that it is frequently under the scrutiny of others who believe they know what is best for both participants. Some of these difficulties have been nicely documented by Shearer (1981) who has examined the mutual handicap of helper and helped; the one unable to ask for help, the other unable to offer it in ways which do not create uneasiness for both. Shearer and Cunningham (1977) have also provided some cogent case material to demonstrate the way in which help can force disabled people into invalidism and the resentment thereby created in those robbed of their remaining independence. But even where the helper and the helped have developed an understanding of their own, it may be challenged by people who are not party to the arrangement and can increase the uncertainty of the provider.

Mrs W and her husband had developed a relationship which allowed her to retain a degree of independence, and Mrs O and her family had a similar arrangement which sometimes had to be protected from modification by outsiders.

Mrs W: I think it's wrong to have people wait on you. I've got a thing about that I don't like people waiting on me for every little thing. Now my husband he comes in and he'll have his cup of tea and I'll go into the kitchen and he'll call out 'Bring me another one in!' I've got to bring that tea into him. He doesn't treat me as though you know, 'I'll do it. I'll get it for you.' He calls out 'Bring me another.' I think it helps an awful lot because I want to do these things. If you wait on a disabled person for every little thing it makes them an imbecile. My husband doesn't treat me as an invalid, he calls out if he wants anything. Or he'll say to me, you see I do all the washing up, he'll say 'Haven't you done that yet?'

Mrs O: My family are very good. You see, now this old lady who visits me, her daughter would have got on my nerves because she was always very kind but . . . I know it's awful to say she would have got on my nerves, but she wanted to do everything. Well my family . . . people might think . . . well I know people think they're a bit cruel but they're not. They know if I want help I'll ask for it. So my husband will get out of the car and open the door for me but he won't do anything else unless I ask. Well, I know a lot of people think he should help her out but I want to do it on my own and it's the same with my daughters, as somebody said to her the other day, 'Go on, help your mother.' And she said 'My mother knows whether she wants help or not,' like that, you see, well they might think . . . but it's not the right way to go on for me. If they'd have fussed over me I'd be stuck in a chair doing nothing.

Comments by outsiders concerning the amount of help requested by a disabled person and the amount of help given by the one providing care can create feelings of guilt in both; one may feel he or she is asking for too much and the other that he or she is giving too little. With a fluctuating condition like rheumatoid arthritis, the dividing line between necessary and disabling assistance may be a very difficult one to draw so that helpers face the constant dilemma of not knowing whether they are expecting or giving too much. This dilemma became more acute when outsiders offered contradictory opinions. Certainly, Mrs R's daughter felt this was a factor contributing to the temporary breakdown of their relationship.

> *Carol:* People were coming to me and saying I shouldn't let her do this and I shouldn't let her do that and on the one hand I had the doctor saying I should and on the other all these people saying to me 'you shouldn't, you're really pushing her too hard' and, you know, 'it'll be your fault,' so I was tending to smother, wasn't I?

An equally difficult problem for family or friends to come to terms with is their inability to help, when the practical assistance they can give does little to reduce the person's suffering. Mrs G's main problem was pain and limited mobility and, consequently, there was nothing her sons and daughter could really do to make things better. She sensed this caused them pain and had stopped asking them to visit.

> *Mrs G:* I think it's the helplessness that makes them sad. If I had a cut arm they would say 'Right, mum, we'll bandage it for you and we'll look after it and do this and that until you're better.' But I can sense this helplessness feeling and it makes them sort of embarrassed or withdrawn or shall I say they don't seem to be able to cope psychologically with a situation they can't do much about. That's from their side and from my side . . . I don't even sort of say to my children 'Come. . . .'

Because dependency on others can increase the disabled person's sense of abnormality, both parties to the relationship would often strive to reduce the amount of help needed or given. Some of the respondents would simply refuse help and insist on doing things themselves despite the cost in terms of pain; Mrs J was a good example of this. Others would attempt to educate friends and new acquaintances so that the help they gave was indeed useful, and some would try to get access to resources which would reduce the dependence of one person or another. At the time of the interviewing Mrs D had to be lifted in and out of the bath by her husband. He was more than willing to continue to do this but thought it better for his wife to be able to manage by herself. They were planning to remove the bath and install a shower because, 'She's no need to be dependent on me, she can do things on her own if indeed we had the things to help her.' Aids and adaptations, like money, have the capacity to transform social relations.

Social support and social networks

While most chronically sick and disabled persons receive most of their help from spouses and daughters (Moroney 1976), it is also the case that helper and helped exist within wider social networks which may be more or less supportive. Among this group of people the extent and composition of their networks varied as did the extent and nature of the support received. On the one hand, Mrs J had an extensive network of relatives all living within her part of London, which included three brothers and two sisters and their families and a number of aunts and uncles who were still alive and considered very much part of the family. In fact, Mrs J's network consisted entirely of family, and anyone else was regarded as a stranger. In contrast, Mrs A had no living relatives apart from her mother, and neither did her husband, but both had a large network of very helpful friends made through their involvement with a local church. At the other extreme were Mr H and his wife and Mr M, who, through accidents of personal history, had no relatives and whose friendship networks did not seem to have stood the test of their increasing disability.

Only a small proportion of those with relatively extensive networks were in receipt of much in the way of practical help, though all derived a great deal of comfort from the knowledge that there was such a resource on which they could call at times of crisis. Again, at one end of the spectrum were Mr S and his wife who were so well integrated into a network of relatives that a prolonged illness in Mrs S had not given rise to any additional problems.

Mr S: We always see the family, they come round here or we go up there. There's always somebody in here, we're never on our own. They mix in, they don't look on her as an outcast 'cus I can't do what they do. If ever there's anything we want, if we're in trouble, we ring up and they're over, you know, no bother like that. If anything goes wrong with the car I ring the wife's brother up so I've got no worries or anything like that. When my wife was ill her mother came over and helped out so I had no worry there. My daughter used to come, my son would come down, we never had a problem like, 'cus we've got a good family, they're always helpful.

At the other end of the spectrum perhaps was Mrs V, whose two sons and families lived on the same street but rarely called to see her: 'We're not very clannish, never have been. I'm here all the time, I never get asked anywhere, I don't mind.' Nevertheless, when she suffered a fall in the garden and had to be taken to hospital, the family did rally round and help in whatever way they could. In some respects her situation differed from that of those without relatives who received no help other than that given by social service personnel.

One reason why wider family and friendship networks did not provide much in the way of help was that they were not asked to do so. Either there was no need for additional help, or the family and friends that existed were not sufficiently close emotionally, or the respondents did not feel that it was appropriate to seek help from people who had families and responsibilities of their own. While Mr and Mrs I could have been helped in a number of ways, they received little direct support from their respective families.

> *Mrs I:* I'm not very close to my family, you know what I mean, so I don't really keep in contact with them. I don't see them a lot . . . our upbringing wasn't very. . . . My mother sometimes gets a fit in her head and comes down and sees us. His family are close but I haven't been running to them. I could have but I haven't like, you know. They've got families of their own to bring up. His brothers have both got three or four kiddies. You can't expect them to keep running round for us all the time.

For a time Mrs I had had an arrangement with the young woman next door who was at home expecting her first child; Mrs I would do her shopping and in return she would sit with Mr I or keep popping in and out to check that he was all right. In that way Mrs I could manage to do her own shopping, go to collect the family's allowances from the post office, or do anything else that took her out of the house. This arrangement had come to an end following the birth of the neighbour's child: 'I wouldn't ask her now, it wouldn't be fair to her. I mean, she's got a family of her own to bring up.'

Mrs G lost her entire family during the war, and her late husband had little family either, so despite having four children there was no one on whom Mrs G could call.

> *Mrs G:* Obviously I've got no family, I have children, that's different. My husband had a sister I met once and I don't know what her

surname is. You see, not only do I not have any family, my children haven't either. They've grown up without grandads and grandmas and uncles and aunts, something they found hard to understand. It's only my grandchildren will have uncles and aunts. That was the thinking behind having four 'cus I thought 'Well, if everything else fails they'll have each other.' So although I've got four children and four grandchildren you couldn't exactly say I could make the children look after me. They're too young, say, in twenty years time, yes. Everybody's saying why don't you make the children do this that and the other, well this sort of thing doesn't happen until you're usually 70 and it happened to me at 50. I keep saying that to different social workers who say 'Can't your children?' I say 'They're looking after each other.' That's all they've got, they can't take on a mum as well, 'cus they're still in their twenties and trying to put their first home together and you can't push 'em. At least I don't think you can. How much pressure can you put on them? You can't, it's nonsense.

It is not possible using the kind of data employed in this study to determine the extent to which an absence of social networks can be attributed to chronic illness and disability or vice versa. There are questions which require large samples and fairly sophisticated designs if they are to be answered with any certainty. Clearly, there are a number of factors at work shaping the extent and character of social networks and chronic illness is but one. However, some social networks do seem to fragment following the onset of appreciable disability, and with them potential sources of help, and one or two good illustrations of this were found among the respondents. If it happened, it seemed to happen fairly rapidly and left those affected bitter and confused:

Mr H: Since we've been here not a friend has offered to come and help, no one's come round, she's had to struggle with it all herself. You see, they say 'I'm sorry, old boy, but I'm off to America next week' or 'I'm sorry, I'm working every night.' It's amazing how people suddenly evaporate. But when I was well I used to go round and help people decorate, cut their lawns, do their shopping but I find none of this. I don't think there was a weekend we weren't out in the car with someone or round someone's place. And they never come and say 'Can we get you a loaf of bread or anything else?' People we used to wine and dine before I was ill. No, they've just gone like a puff of smoke. Oh yes, when they could come and wine and dine and come out in the car it was great but it gradually fizzled out they gradually came less and less. And anything to do. . . . You see, if you said 'Could you put a curtain rod up there?' 'Oh yes, we'll try and come next week,' and next week, of course, they don't come. It's been a bit of a surprise to me. From what I can see they're a dead loss.

From the accounts provided by the respondents, this breakdown in social networks was sometimes the result of a process in which they withdrew and sometimes the product of the withdrawal of others. Just as they may withdraw from their family when in severe pain, these people sometimes withdrew from their wider circle of contacts, but for different reasons and usually more permanently. One reason was that the relationship between the respondents and their friends became strained particularly at times when they were very incapacitated.

> *Mrs A:* I did go through a period, I think a lot of arthritics have gone through this at times, of resentment against one's fitter friends when they trot in and tell you what they've been doing you feel a little envious and a bit put out. I went through a stage like this when I must have been beastly to be friendly with, in fact I used to avoid them, because I resented everything.

Where the withdrawal came from the other side it largely seemed to happen because the disabled person could no longer share in activities that their friends took for granted; the old pattern could not be maintained or could only be maintained at too great a cost.

> *Mr H:* It's amazing how quickly you lose your patience. Believe you me, I lost all of my friends. Oh yes, people who used to come round and say 'Now look, let's go out in the car, let's go down to the coast.' Not any more. They only do it once and then they find they've got a job to lift me in and out of the car and they've got to fold the wheelchair up and put it back in the car and then they've got to get me out and when they get somewhere they can't go wandering through the woods and the fields because of the chair so they don't do it twice. You see if they're parents of kids it rather spoils it to take a chair 'cus you can't go here and you can't go there. And they can't say 'Let's go out to the pub and have a glass and so on.' And if you go to a restaurant they've got the problem of getting in there and getting the wheelchair up to the table, and any friend we do have they get embarrassed because they see I can't get the food up to my mouth and the wife says, you know, 'I'll do it for you' and I think they think 'Well, one or two people in the restaurant are looking, poor man,' you see. I think they find that a bit embarrassing. I think that's the reason people tend to drop away.

Other respondents lost supportive networks when they moved house or when redevelopment of their street dispersed people on whom they used to rely. Mrs V had been part of a long-standing network of neighbours who had raised families together and had continued to help each other after the children were grown. The network had fragmented when many of the houses on the street were emptied for renovation and young people moved in with whom Mrs V had little in common. Once lost, such supportive networks were difficult to replace; Mrs V never got out of the house so rarely saw her new neighbours. Some of those who have moved discovered that their flats and houses had been constructed with privacy in mind so never saw or came into contact with the people living next door. The only one who had been successful in developing a new group of friends was Mrs G who, though Jewish, had a number of what she called 'church friends': 'I know you've probably never met a Hebrew Christian but, you see, I think I needed something to hang on to that was rather stronger than myself and this is how it came about.' Because limited mobility and lack of participation in community affairs made it difficult to make new friends, Mrs O and her husband had finally decided not to move to a house that might be more conveniently constructed but would remain in an area where they knew everyone and could count on some support if anything should happen to one or the other.

Marriage and family life

It is now common for helping professionals or others who have dealings with chronically sick people to talk about 'the disabled family' in recognition of the fact that the effects of a long-term illness extend beyond the individual afflicted to envelop their close associates (Blaxter 1976). While disability 'disables the normal' by rendering the rules of social interaction inapplicable, it also has longer term effects on others, particularly family members, whose daily lives may be severely dislocated by the presence of a disabled person in the household. These effects, both on family members and between family members, have tended to concentrate on the impact of mental illness (Yarrow, Clausen, and Robbins 1955; Mills 1962, Sainsbury and Grad de Alarcon 1974; Creer and Wing 1974), and there is little comparable data with respect to long-term physical illness, at least with regard to the disabled adult.

Some of the effects of disability on others have been touched on in the preceding chapters which have offered a glimpse of reduced opportunities for employment and leisure, the development of social isolation, poverty, and stigma. Within this group disability also had an impact on health. A combination of poor housing conditions and the physical and emotional strain of caring for a disabled spouse had proved too much for some of the wives.

Mrs I: It's just bringing me down. I had to go to the doctor 'cus I was on Valium, it was just pulling me down. He used to say 'I want a bath.' I used to dread it, you know. 'I think I'll have a bath now.' 'Oh no.' In the end I was wishing he wouldn't get in the bath 'cus he was that heavy to get in and out. I'm only seven stone and I was lifting him in and out, it's just not on. I said to the rehab woman 'I'm going to break one day and what's he going to do then?'

Mr H was so concerned about the impact of his disability on his wife's life in general and health in particular that he had begun to consider the possibility of going into residential care.

> *Mr H:* We've got to face things, they're just going from bad to worse. It may be better if I'm in a proper State home because there's no life for her with this waiting on me hand and foot and day and night. It's no life for her a woman of her age. So we've thought of this, but we've been married for 34 years which is a long time and the whole thing has distressed us very much.

Like many others in the same situation the problem here was how to give Mrs H a break from her caring role. The nursing unit attached to their block of flats closed at five o'clock so there was no possibility of Mrs H getting out in the evening. Nor did there seem to be much of a possibility that she could get away for a short holiday, if she would go alone that is, since they knew of no institution that would admit him temporarily to relieve her stress. His own experience led him to reflect on stories he had been told of similarly disabled people abandoned by their relatives and admitted to residential care: 'I can understand it because people do have their own lives to lead, you can't expect someone to hang around for ten or twenty years because you're in a wheelchair.' He and his wife were learning how difficult it was for someone to live his or her own life and care for a disabled person without help.

According to this group of respondents, one of the commonest problems encountered in terms of family relationships was the development of friction between themselves and other members of the family, most usually those living within the household. The widowed, in looking back, recalled that conflict was a feature of their domestic existence, and the single also recalled similar experiences when they lived with family. Data has been presented in this and other chapters which shows that such discord may arise for a number of reasons. Problems of legitimacy and dependency were obvious sources of strain and so was the decline in standards when tasks were eventually handed over to already over-burdened family members. However, the most frequent type of friction they encountered was that associated with pain. All said that at times pain made them irritable, bad tempered, unreasonable, and intolerant so that small matters became blown up out of all proportion and gave rise to bitter arguments and the like. At the first interview Mr F was in severe pain and having a difficult time with his family.

> *Mr F:* I get short tempered with the boy if he gets all his things out and they get all over the place and I can't get my feet over the damn things. You do get short tempered, you pick up people's remarks, somebody

makes a small remark and you're liable to jump at them whereas before you'd take it as a joke . . . it's hard to take jokes. Little things get on your nerves, things you wouldn't usually take notice of you lose your temper. I'm not keen on people coming in. The wife's relatives, if they come, I sit for a while then make an excuse and go to bed. I can't explain it, I just know I'm going to end up in a temper. I prefer to get out of the way rather than cause an argument.

One year later, when pain levels had subsided and family relationships were restored, Mr F looked back and elaborated further on the problems they experienced.

Int: Last time you said you got irritated with the family. . . . Has that changed?

Mr F: Oh, it has, yes. You know, I think they used to try and do too much for me and try and help all the time and all you want is to be left alone and suffer alone, you know. You don't want people going around you and messing about, making you comfortable and the worst thing that can be done, you know, is people standing around talking, that used to get on my nerves all the time, or a television on, that used to get on my nerves. All I wanted to do really was to be left alone. I used to spend more time really sitting in the kitchen on hard chairs rather than sit here listening to the television and listening to the children. But I used to give them a dog's life, you know, but not now.

Int: Do you think they could ever tell when you were in pain?

Mr F: Oh yes, they used to keep out of my way. But as I say, they probably didn't mean it, they were probably doing it to try and help, you know, but they were upsetting me more than if, you know. If they had left me alone everything would have been all right.

Int: What did they try and do?

Mr F: Well, especially in the winter, this is old property, and it does get bitterly cold sometimes. Well, as you can see, I've got three fires in here I've been using all winter and they'd go up and get blankets and pillows, you know, you wouldn't want to lie down but in the end you'd have to lie down just to keep the peace with them, you know, and get away from them making cups of tea and things like that. You know, they'd say 'Do you want a cup of tea?' and you say 'No' and a couple of minutes later 'Do you want a cup of tea?' You lose your temper answering the same question three or four times. But they were only trying to help in their own way but I used to get the needle with them. It used to upset me but it was probably me, I was just bad tempered at the time that's the truth of the matter. It got to the stage really where they were glad to get out of the house in the morning and they were dreading coming back at night 'cus I was here. But it's all changed now, we go out together now.

These problems were not confined to acute flare-ups, though conflict may be particularly marked at these times, but continued throughout the illness career. Mrs X found that even after 20 years of living with pain she was still a little difficult.

> *Mrs X:* I'm inclined to be very short with people, very short. I don't care what anybody says it makes you terribly bad tempered. It really does. I used to treat my husband rotten . . . if the children did anything to upset me I used to vent all my spite on him. It wasn't very nice for him but he stuck it. It's the continual pain, it can't be anything else.

Over time, the families of the respondents seemed to be able to come to terms with this kind of conflict, accepting it as a fact of life and developing ways of managing or neutralizing it. Mr T had a way of coping with Mrs T's bad moods and Mr W would often be able to defuse Mrs W's temper.

> *Mrs T:* I get very irritable with my husband and I'm not at all proud of having to admit that. Let me separate it properly . . . we have the normal disagreements that any married couple will have because we're both of us strong characters and we both have strong views on many things and if those views don't tie up we have an argument as any married couple will do and then we might go on to say one or two silly things and then one of us will always say, even though it might not be said with good grace, 'I'm sorry, I shouldn't have said that' and the other one usually with equally bad grace will say 'All right, it's my fault.' Now, that's one thing but when I become irritable with the pain this is something else again. I can be totally unreasonable and am from time to time, totally unreasonable, and he will never take me up, rather than do that he will go out of the room and leave me for two or three minutes and when he comes back in I'll start off again but he will never pick up the gauntlet under those circumstances and what he does is give me enough time to, sort of, vent my irritation and then come over and put his arms round me and that normally finishes up with me having a bit of a grizzle and then it's all right. But I'm very ashamed of that aspect . . . I do try and control it because frankly I think he deserves better and the next day I start going through it and I think 'You fool, what the hell's the matter with you behaving in that way?' but it's no good giving yourself a lecture afterwards.

> *Mrs W:* I get that bad tempered when I'm in pain. My poor husband usually gets the back end of that because if I get a lot of pain and something he'll say I'll contradict him and I'll argue, I'll be that way with it. He understands, he knows me. He's a great one because the other night I couldn't get my feet into bed and as he tipped my feet he got them caught in his pyjama bottom and I said 'I wish you'd watch what you're doing you've hurt my toe.' And he laughs at me and that

makes me laugh. So I said 'I don't think there's anything funny.' And he said 'There is, your face,' and with this laughing it goes. But I do get very niggly.

Despite the fact that these kind of conflicts are tied to pain, the respondents concerned could not entirely absolve themselves of responsibility for the strains imposed on their relationships with other members of the family; it was their fault; they ought to be more patient and more able to control their temper. This only served to heighten their guilt, for it was one further example of the way the illness and its effects impinged on the quality of life of their close associates.

The mechanisms that families employ for containing conflict do sometimes fail, and major disputes occur which cause significant rifts in family relationships. During the course of her voluntary work with disabled people, Mrs R had seen this many times and was well aware how easily an ordinary domestic dispute could develop a momentum of its own with tragic consequences simply because the right kind of help was not available at the right time. At those times when the family could not accommodate or resolve conflict, an intermediary was required who could come in at short notice and help restore the status quo. Mrs R and her daughter rarely quarrelled but when they did, 'It's really awful, it's terrible, I say really nasty things.' She was well aware of how unreasonable and stubborn she could be at times and recognized these as danger points when outside help was desperately needed: 'There should be someone there that you can turn to, even if it's only for an hour or two hours. They could, sort of, smooth things over a little bit because it happens in every home.' Soon after the second interview 'an ordinary domestic dispute' fuelled rather than resolved by the intervention of others led to Mrs R's daughter leaving home and a series of experiences Mrs R later described as 'a nightmare'. These included admission to a residential home, five weeks of coping alone, and a short stay in hospital following an overdose. Mrs R's account, given at a third interview, is reproduced in some detail in the next chapter.

The studies by Sainsbury (1970), Topliss (1979), and Blaxter (1976) suggest that marriages are at risk following the onset of disability in one partner, the breakdown happening soon after onset rather than after a long period of strain. The first two found a higher incidence of breakdown where the woman became disabled, while the last found the reverse. The small group of individuals interviewed in this study cannot be used to enlarge upon these findings, nor can they be used to say much about the chances of disabled people finding a partner. In fact, the people interviewed presented a complex pattern. One quarter of the group, three women and three men, were single though in most cases there was little to suggest that disability had reduced their chances of marriage. Most had suffered onset relatively late in life after many years of singlehood. In fact, five people had married or started to cohabit after onset, three of these when their disability was severe. The remainder of the respondents were or had been married, and where breakdown had occurred this was mostly through the death of one partner. In only two cases had marital separation occurred. Mrs R had been married and divorced twice and her disability seemed to be of relevance in both instances. Mrs D had left her husband because his gambling and stealing were having an adverse effect on her arthritis. There is no way of telling whether or not things might have been different if she had not been chronically ill. If a general picture emerges at all it is that marriages seemed to survive, though that might have been due to the particular personalities involved and the circumstances in which they found themselves.

> *Mrs W:* I think deep down what has always worried me is that I've not been able to do the things with him that I should normally have done. To go out and about a lot, you know. I'm lucky in some senses I suppose, he's a very quiet person, likes his home, likes his car, he doesn't drink, happy to go out and sit in the sun with a book, that sort of man he is. I suppose he's a lot quieter than I am 'cus I love discos and parties. I'll still go now. He's rather reserved. He'll say sometimes 'I don't want to go, you go', or he'll take me and leave me with friends and collect me later. But what's always worried me is I've never been able to say 'Oh, come on, let's go here, let's go there.' And I've often wondered whether that's kept him in. But he never seems to worry, he never moans about anything. Some peole have said to me 'It's not much of a life for him', and I say 'Well, no, but then he can go out if he wants to.' I don't say 'You can't. You've got to stop with me.' But he never does, he never wants to go anywhere.

> *Mrs X:* I couldn't bear my husband near me, I screamed blue murder if he came near me. How I got pregnant the last twice I really don't know. But, Oh no, I used to lay down the law.
> *Int:* Did that affect the way you got on with your husband?
> *Mrs X:* He worshipped the ground I walked on. But let me tell you this, my husband was twenty years older than me which makes all the difference. I think had I had a younger man he would have walked out on me.

As Mrs X suggests, age may have been an important factor in explaining the success of some of these marriages since many respondents did not become appreciably disabled until quite late on in their marital career when social and physical activity would have been expected to decline anyway. This is not wholly borne out by the data, or at least not by the accounts of the two respondents who talked at length about the physical side of their marriage; the absence of a sexual relationship was not something which had been anticipated but something to which the partners had had to adjust.

Mr K: Physically my wife and I have not been able to do the normal things of married life for a long time. Well, I'd be a fine sort of bloke if I went out and dragged other women in but that happens with a lot of cases. It causes a great deal of distress . . . I mean, imagine living with your wife for all these numbers of years when you've been young and had a family and you've made love and all of a sudden it stops just like that. How do you think people adjust . . . I mean, you've got to adjust it's part of your job to adjust. I couldn't desert her. I mean, she needs me more now than she ever did. It's no good sitting down and crying into your beer. We manage to get by, we spend all our time together. She knows I wouldn't hurt her, there's no reason to, she's still the same girl I married. I've accepted it . . . it's there to be accepted. You marry a woman for better or worse and if anything happens to one of the partners it's up to the other to muck in.

Mr K had been helped to adjust by a particular set of circumstances. During his wife's disability he had suffered two coronaries, the last one so severe the hospital had telephoned his wife to say he was not expected to survive: 'But some power got me going again and here I am, it's now my job to look after her. This is why I think I was given a second chance. Since I've had spiritual guidance I know I'm doing the right thing.'

Although she did not marry until the age of 39, Mrs T wanted to have children and so did her husband since none had been produced in his previous two marriages. This had proved to be impossible; because of her difficulty they had not been able to consummate the marriage. They had briefly considered approaching their doctor to see if an operation would make a physical relationship possible but Mr T had decided against that because of the risks and pain involved. His view had been one of 'let's accept all the other good things we've got together, make the best of those, regret the fact but at the same time not take it out of context'. Subsequently, Mr T had worked very hard to make Mrs T accept there was no question of blame and was largely, but not entirely, successful:

Mrs T: I suppose now that I'm talking about it there's still that tiny little gnaw at the back of my mind saying 'It's your fault, you're not able to fulfil, not the most important part of our life together, but a basic and important one nonetheless.' It's taken a tremendous amount of mental adjustment.

Mrs T was, however able to find advantage in disadvantage, and felt their early years together had been easier than they might: their big problem had overshadowed all the other ordinary problems of adjustment that two people in their forties setting up home together inevitably confront. Fifteen years later she was able to write in a letter sent just prior to the first interview: 'I can hardly do a thing here. And he treats me like a Goddess. I'm a very lucky woman and a very happy one.'

Not all relationships were so supportive. Mrs G and Mrs R both had unhappy marriages, the former ending with the death of her husband, the latter in separation and divorce. While Mrs R attributed both the marriage and the separation to her disability, it was not altogether clear that Mrs G's marriage would have been much better had she not become chronically ill. However both of their stories offer a modicum of support for the hypothesis that marriages fail when disability or the response to disability in one partner prevents fulfilment of the needs of the other or where both are unable to adjust their needs in line with new realities. Mrs G received little support from her husband throughout a long and unhappy marriage; she had continued to work during her illness and had been left with sole responsibility for the care of their four children.

> *Mrs G:* You see, he learned that the only way to get attention was to get sick, so when I got sick he wouldn't have that as we were diverting attention from him to me. Being rather a wild gentleman it wasn't too good a trip. So when he departed this life I just breathed a sigh of relief. You see, had I been home here, had somebody to go home to I probably would have taken my kids and gone home. He used to bring tension in and out with him into the house and with that tension gone we could all now relax and this is how it is to this day. Now we're a family.

Soon after her first marriage broke up, Mrs R married for a second time. Her first husband had wanted her to go back to him but she felt that it would never work: 'He'd always travelled, he was a traveller and I thought "Well, I can't travel with him and he'll never give up" and that's how it broke up. It was my fault really 'cus I couldn't live up to him.' This second marriage turned out to be 'the biggest mistake of my life,' and looking back Mrs R said 'I wouldn't have looked at him twice had I been fit and healthy. He wasn't my type of person.' In the early days the marriage worked well, despite the fact that Mrs R was bed-ridden for much of the time and her new husband had to take over the management of the household.

> *Mrs R:* In that first year he was very good. He used to come home and cook and afterwards he said 'The happiest days of my life were when I used to come home and have to do the cooking and iron the kid's clothes.' He used to say 'You're too independent.' In fact, the last thing he said to me was 'You're too independent.' He said 'Had you broken down a few times . . . .' Perhaps I was wrong there, you can be too

independent. I remember one time I thought 'I'll get up tonight and cook dinner' and it was such an effort and I was so pleased with myself even though it was only a simple meal. And when he came in he was like a child, he just sulked, you know, it's unbelievable but there are men that have to be needed I suppose.

Subsequently, other problems developed which eventually led to the breakdown of the marriage, separation, and divorce. Again, Mrs R attributed these problems to her disability.

Mrs R: For the first year he'd do anything for me but when he found I couldn't go out with him . . . that was when I was walking a bit, it was agony but he didn't know, but as I got worse and couldn't go out with him that was when things started to go a bit. . . . He would go out and come back late and there was nothing I could do about it. I used to dread him coming home from work because I'd think 'If I don't go with him he's going drinking and he's going to come back paralytic.' I just couldn't live up to him, you can't keep saying 'I've got pain here, I've got pain there.' It's got to be a very understanding person to understand this complaint especially then 'cus my hands weren't deformed as they are now. So I had to put up with it until I retaliated and he came back and found I wasn't there. I'd managed to get to the person upstairs and I pretended I'd been out on the razzle. He was so shocked. It was all pretence, you had to put these things on, it was so stupid. But it was very hard trying to live a normal married life when you are disabled.

Because rheumatoid arthritis involves severe pain as well as disability it seemed to have a profound effect on parenting and the parental role. All the respondents with children had found parenthood problematic in one respect or another and a major source of worry and distress. The problems sometimes began in pregnancy and were often created by the responses of others who assume that disability and pregnancy do not go together (Campling 1981).

Mrs R: When I had Carol I felt like a criminal 'cus at antenatal I'd drop my stick or something stupid and I'd think 'What have I let myself in for? Should I have done this?' I wanted her because it was my second husband, you see. And then people frightened me, they used to say 'Well, you'll have to have a sling,' and I thought 'God!', and they said 'Well, you won't be able to manage her' and then they said 'Of course, you'll have to have a Caesarean.' So, of course, I used to get panicky. 'What on earth's happening? What have I done?' Well, when I did have her I had no trouble at all. I enjoyed her babyhood. I bought the biggest pram you ever saw so I could lean on it and I enjoyed her childhood more than the others.

The only problem Mrs R was able to recall was again created by the responses of others; she felt that her adequacy as a parent was constantly questioned.

> *Mrs R:* They thought at school until I went and saw them that because she'd got a disabled mother she had to do everything in the house which wasn't so 'cus I was doing it myself then and the limit was when Carol had a pain in her leg and they said 'Had she been scrubbing floors?' Well, she never did things like that at that age.

Some of the women did find motherhood highly problematic and would not have been able to cope had they not had the support of family and friends. Mrs X suffered her first big attack when the youngest of her four children was three months old and the eldest eight years. These early years were very difficult despite the fact that there were a number of people who came to help. Her mother came every day to clean the house, do the laundry, and cook for the children. Her sister-in-law would take the children for weekends and take them away on holiday, and for the six months following her first discharge from hospital the care of the baby was shared between her sister-in-law and a friend. They took it in turn to have the child with them for spells of fourteen days. However, there were other problems which were not so easily solved.

> *Mrs X:* My hands were so painful I couldn't bear any of my children to touch me. I couldn't cuddle them, my hands and arms were too painful and I hardly dare have any of them come near me. I missed out on a lot. And, of course, my temper was very short, I was inclined to give a smack whereas had I been in perfect health I wouldn't have done. It affected me terrible, I had no time to reason with the children, no time to sit down and . . . I suppose I was in such pain I didn't have the patience with them. I'm surprised they turned out so well. I never enjoyed my children. Shall I put it that way? I was in such pain I never really enjoyed them.

Mrs G's problems were perhaps more acute if only because she had no network on whom she was able to call in a crisis. Her husband refused to take care of the children during her many spells in hospital, and she sometimes had to discharge herself early because he would not go to the trouble of having them taken into care. It was for this reason she said 'When I knew I was ill I thought "Heaven, give me ten years to bring up the children." ' Her children's early years were frequently disrupted by admission to residential care, 'I think they've seen the inside of every children's home in Surrey', and their education suffered by continual changes of schools.

Mrs G: It didn't just damage me, it damaged them as well. As my eldest said to me 'We're all damaged, we're all affected.'

Now that she was a grandparent Mrs G still encountered problems: 'How do you explain to a three-year old they can't climb up your legs or dump all their toys in your lap?'

It was not only the women who experienced problems in parenting; fulfilling a parental role was also problematic for the men. Their concern was largely confined to their inability to share activities with their children which had to be abandoned or given over to others. These problems were particularly acute when the children were too young to understand their father's disability or where attempts had been made to conceal the extent of the illness from them.

Mr S: I've never given my son no pleasure, many a time he's said to the wife 'Why don't daddy come swimming? Why don't he play football?' You know, when he didn't understand. What happens is the wife does all that, she takes him swimming, she plays tennis with him, what I couldn't do she does for him. You know, he's said a few times, why don't I help and play in the games. I used to feel choked like, seeing them all go off swimming and I'm stuck here waiting for 'em to get back.

An inability to participate in these kinds of activities not only excludes the disabled person from one face of family life but effectively underlines the extent of his or her limitation. It is for this reason that requests from children for outings and the like can give rise to some distress. Mr F said 'They couldn't understand why we couldn't go camping and everything else and he'd ask "Can we go?" and in the end it used to upset me to think that I couldn't.' Some of these problems were resolved as children grew up and began to understand the meaning of parental illness. They ceased to be such a problem in the later years simply because children became independent and no longer expected parents to participate in all of their activities. Nevertheless, chronic illness in one parent can still act as a constraint, particularly so where certain kinds of resources are in short supply. For the I's the problem was one of a lack of physical space.

Mrs I: The children like to bring their friends in and if he's not well, you can't have all that noise and that. If we had an upstairs when they're in they'd be out of the way but on one level you can't. In the end I had to pack my daughter's record player away 'cus it was disturbing him. I said 'I'm packing it in case we move.' You know, just so's the kid couldn't play it. It's not fair on the children having to keep telling them they can't do things, they're going to say they can't have nobody in, any kid is going to say it.

While many chronically sick people believe they are a burden on their family, some of this data gives rise to the impression that the family, and the needs of its individual members, imposes a significant burden on those with a long-term illness. Families can be a tremendous advantage in helping someone to cope with disability, both in a practical and emotional sense, but they can at times constitute a disadvantage. This is the case even when relationships within the family are positive and supportive, for the presence of others can act as a constraint on individual choice. As Miss L said, reviewing her own situation, 'At least I'm single. I can be selfish up to a point. Some people just have to put on a front for their family, they just can't decide to go to bed if they've got children. Some are like little old ladies and they're only forty.' Obligations and responsibilities do not cease following the onset of illness and disability; they just become more difficult to discharge.

7 *The welfare bureaucracy*

Medicine is one of two major institutions to which chronically sick and disabled persons turn for help; the other is the bureaucracy of the welfare state. The former helps to control the disease and its more immediate effects, the latter to mitigate the wider social and economic consequences of the disease and the disability it produces. It is this welfare bureaucracy, consisting of a complex and confusing system of social and economic provision, which is responsible for reducing the disadvantage originating in long-term disabling illness. Consequently, a number of organizations and services have been developed in order to manage problems of employment, housing, income, education, and rehabilitation encountered by disabled people. It is clear that existing provision falls far short of its goal of meeting the needs of those it aims to help; the categories with which the system operates do not match the needs of those to whom they are applied, provision is fundamentally unjust creating artificial divisions between people with the same needs and, in some respects, it perpetuates the disadvantage of those who have little choice but to rely on it for help (Walker 1980). The main problem is that existing services were not developed on the basis of a coherent understanding of the origins and consequences of disability but emerged in piecemeal fashion in response to historical contingency and political pressure. Inevitably, they reflect and are limited by wider social values and attitudes towards social welfare (Topliss 1975). This is not to deny the enormous benefits that disabled individuals have derived from this system of provision. Equally clearly, they would be far worse off if it did not exist. Nevertheless, current policies and practices are grossly inadequate to secure the integration and participation of disabled people in all aspects of community life.

Discussions of the origins and limitations of welfare services abound, and there is no need to summarize or enlarge upon them here. Nor is there any need to examine in detail the gap between the self-defined needs of chronically sick people and the services available to meet them since that has been admirably covered elsewhere (Blaxter 1976). This chapter has a far more limited aim and seeks to examine the experiences of the twenty-four people interviewed in dealing with the services and organizations intended to promote their well-being. The main issue discussed is the way these services and organizations may create as many problems as they solve.

Getting into the system

Getting into the welfare system is a haphazard process and is more often the result of informal rather than formal referral mechanisms. Knowledge and information concerning benefits and services are just as likely to be supplied by friends, acquaintances, and fellow sufferers as they are by the professionals involved in health and welfare. While the majority of the respondents had received advice and help from representatives of welfare agencies at some stage in their career, this rarely followed automatically from their contacts with medical care. Even those most recently disabled and hospitalized had not been referred to a social worker. While Mr I was in hospital, it was suggested that he might like to see 'an almoner', but nothing had been arranged by the time he was discharged. Nor had he been referred at any of his out-patient appointments despite the fact that a social worker was attached to the Rheumatology Department in which he was treated and had an office adjacent to the clinic. He had been unemployed for two years before he contacted a social worker on the advice of a clerk in the local Social Security office, and her main contribution was to refer him on to a rehabilitation officer who then supplied a number of aids and appliances he found very useful. When diagnosed as having multiple sclerosis, Mrs K was advised by her daughter-in-law to join the local Multiple Sclerosis Society. It was then that she was advised to contact a social worker and also told by fellow sufferers about the local branch of the Rheumatism and Arthritis Association, who later proved very helpful in advising her about benefits for which she might apply. Subsequently, she received an attendance allowance and an invalid care allowance as her husband had given up his job in order to care for her.

Being in contact with a social worker was not always an effective means of securing access to available benefits and services since some social workers appeared to be less well informed about entitlements and discretionary payments than their clients. Mr I's main problem was a lack of information about what was available and the proper procedures for applying for financial support. The social worker responsible for his case did not appear to understand the system any better than he, nor did she seem to have made use of the welfare rights officer employed by the Social Services Department to advise social workers about the best package of benefits for their clients.

> *Mr I:* She was a very nice person but we was too young for her, you know what I mean. She didn't know what to say, she used to sit here

and we used to tell her and she used to say 'I've got an old man this' and 'an old gel that' which didn't appeal to us 'cus we weren't interested in her other patients. She did say 'We'll try and get you away on holiday' but she couldn't help with the forms or the entitlements. She didn't understand half the things especially the up-to-date things . . . she couldn't help us with the forms. She came in one day and she says 'I don't think I can help you' and I said 'what help you have done we're grateful.'

In the absence of formal help, Mr and Mrs I were left to their own devices and the informal channels on which they had previously relied. For Mrs I the search for benefits to which they might be entitled was a full-time job.

Mrs I: I've gone through other people telling me, friends and neighbours, 'If you go here you get this.' In the past two years we've done it ourselves, I've been listening to other people, you know, 'My husband's got this' they said, 'I went here, I went there.' So I thought 'If you can get it I can get it,' so I've been, sort of, doing it myself, but it's been such a lot of running about. You know, there's so many different little things isn't there. People say 'Why haven't you got that? Why haven't you put in for that?' You know, you never think about them.

As Blaxter (1976) notes, while these informal referral processes may lead to the acquisition of benefits and services, they are subject to a number of disadvantages. Assuming that the experiences of the I's is not typical, formal referral processes are likely to be more efficient in ensuring that people receive the services to which they are entitled. Mr I only learnt of the existence of the mobility allowance shortly before the first interview, and Mr F, who thought he had no need of a social worker, had only recently been told that he might be eligible for a disabled person's car badge which would allow him to park anywhere and avoid the parking fines he always seemed to collect. Informal sources may also lead people to believe that because they are disabled they are automatically entitled to benefits for which they are not, in fact, eligible, leaving them feeling discontented and hard done by when their application is refused. This was often the case where time and energy had been invested in attempting to secure additional payments. Conversely, they may be told they are not entitled to a benefit which is their right and may delay applying or may not apply at all. Mr F had been told by his informant that even people eligible for a disabled person's car badge had a hard time getting it and had only finally applied when he had been caught in a sudden snow storm when attempting to get to the hospital by public transport. Consequently, it is unlikely that informal channels of information will lead to the most advantageous package of benefits and services being claimed so that people end up being financially worse off than they need to be. Mr I was afraid of applying for the mobility allowance because he thought it might be counted as income and lead to a reduction in the other payments that he claimed. He did not know who to contact to discuss the problem and was hoping the rehabilitation officer would enlighten him when she next called. However, where formal channels are ineffective, as they sometimes are, disabled people have no choice but to gather information from whatever source presents itself and manage as best they can.

Problematic aspects of the welfare bureaucracy

To judge by the accounts of the respondents the welfare bureaucracy is, for the most part, inefficient, inaccessible, inflexible, and unresponsive to their needs. It appeared to them to work in its own way and at its own pace regardless of the urgency of their case or the inconvenience it caused. The whole process seemed to be governed by a system of rules and regulations which were arbitrary or irrational and either prevented access to the resources they required or caused unacceptable delays in provision when their eligibility for a benefit or service was granted. These characteristics gave rise to a great deal in the way of discontent and hostility and, on many occasions, overt conflict between the respondents, their relatives, and those who administer the system. Some had learnt through bitter experience that generating conflict was sometimes the only way of getting the system to respond to their needs.

One source of conflict was competing definitions of need. The definitions built into the regulations determining eligibility for services or benefits did not match the definitions employed by the respondents, and it was often difficult for them to see any sense in the rules governing provision. For example, the I's had been denied financial help with a telephone because 'if you've got children who can go out to the phone for you that's out of the question'. To them, that meant that they had no way of calling for help in an emergency: 'You try getting a phone round here at night. They're all smashed up. If anything happened in the middle of the night I wouldn't know where to go.' Similarly, they received what they considered to be inadequate help with their children's clothing.

> *Mrs I:* When I applied for that children's clothing allowance 'cus my son needed trousers she said 'You had one two years ago you can't reapply till September.' He went through a pair of trousers in five weeks. He's just a kid who likes his football and you just can't say to him 'you can't don't ruin them I can't afford another pair.' You can't stop him.
>
> *Mr I:* I mean, all right, they say, well, you get a grant for their school

uniform every two years so their feet mustn't grow for two years. They don't know the out of it, what you've got to pay out. You try rigging two girls out for school, they've got to have uniforms, P.T. gear, swimming gear, winter coats, and summer coats. You try it, it's murder.

Mrs I also found a lack of appreciation of her family's needs on the part of the social security personnel who dealt with her claims for benefits. Her frustration frequently caused her to lose her temper.

Mrs I: Some of them talk out of the back of their head down there. They say *'Why* do you want it? *Why* do you need it? *Why. . . ?'* Well, you wouldn't be down there if you didn't need anything off 'em. I mean if someone was to come here and see what I've got they'd know what I need. I wouldn't have to sit up these places four or five hours and then when I do see somebody lose my temper with them.

Similar conflicts occurred over definitions of eligibility for benefits. Mr M found that the regulations denied him a number of benefits to which he thought he should be entitled. He had been told by the Citizens Advice Bureau that as a disabled person he should be paid a weekly heating allowance, only to discover that his invalidity pension provided him with £5 per week more than the official subsistence level beyond which such additional payments were not made. His disillusionment with the system was exacerbated when he was refused assistance with the cost of travelling to a rehabilitation centre in the West Country to which he had been referred by his doctor, because his income was greater than subsistence level.

Mr M: I said to them 'What you're saying to me is I'm denied medical treatment.' 'No,' they said 'we're not saying that. All we're saying is you've got to pay your own way.' I said 'I can't pay, that's why I've come to you.' You see, you're penalized for working and being diligent. It seems to me if you hadn't worked you'd be entitled to all the things I'm not entitled to 'cus you'd be on a lower rate. But it's morally wrong to me, that is, telling you you cannot have medical treatment and I've worked for my living. There's no justice at all, no way. I'm on a pension and out of work and I don't see why they shouldn't pay it. When you think that a non-contributing person who's never picked up a pen or a shovel can get it and you who've worked and who through no fault of your own, which is a most important point, through no fault of your own you're denied it. That to me is wrong, that to me is not justice.

Mr M's claim for a heating allowance was eventually referred to an Appeals Tribunal and rejected, although he did manage to get to the rehabilitation unit, but only by virtue of the generosity of someone he hardly knew. He had told his story in his local pub and later in the evening someone who had been an acquaintance, but was 'a friend now', had given him an envelope containing sufficient money to pay his fare. To Mr M the system of cash benefits was designed to deny rather than provide for his needs.

> *Mr M:* The rules that are made are very rigid, there's no leeway, the other considerations aren't taken into account. Everything you do, or investigate, or try and do, you find you're not going to get it because you're not so and so and so and so, it's as simple as that. What you're doing all the time is begging. They say you're entitled to it by right and when you ask for it they say you can't have it.

The seeming irrationality of the system, and the extent to which it penalized some of those in genuine need, was reinforced when those administering the system were forced to admit that they could see no logic in the rules governing provision. Mrs I had given up her job in order to take care of her husband and expected to receive an invalid care allowance designed to compensate for loss of earnings through the adoption of a full-time caring role. This allowance is not paid to married and cohabiting women since it was assumed, quite wrongly, that they were likely to be at home occupying a caring role in any event (Coussins 1981) and if caring for a relative other than a husband would be supported financially by their partner. When her claim for the allowance was refused on the grounds she was a married woman residing with her husband, Mrs I appealed against the decision and found the chairman of the Appeals Tribunal equally unable to comprehend the reasoning on which the regulation was based.

> *Mrs I:* If we separated and I had to come and see him everyday they'd pay it, which seems so ridiculous. I can't make it out. Even the chairman of the Tribunal he couldn't make it out. He was baffled. He said to me 'Could you explain it?' and I said 'No, could you explain it to me?' I said 'What they're asking me to do is to leave my husband and then go and visit him everyday 'cus that's what it sounds like.' I said 'I come in quite genuine, I am a respectably married woman and I don't get nothing.' They said 'We'll let you know' and they did let us know and said 'no.'

Mrs I was annoyed at being refused this particular allowance, not only because the rules governing eligibility were without reason, but also because a full-time caring role did prevent her from remaining in paid work. She had always worked to maintain the family income at a reasonable level and like some of the others in the study felt she was being used as a cheap alternative to formal care. The real injustice to which she was subject was exacerbated by perceived injustice and the apparent ability of others to manipulate the system even when they were not in genuine need: 'When you see somebody else getting these things and you know damn well that person goes to work I could scream. Some of these people seem to have such a lot done for them.'

One cash payment which gave rise to a great deal of discontent was the mobility allowance. Probably because mobility was essential to their quality of life, the majority of the respondents had attempted to acquire the allowance, but given the stringency of the regulations governing provision, the majority had been refused. They were left thoroughly dissatisfied for one of two reasons. Firstly, the allowance was designed to promote mobility around the community yet eligibility was determined on the basis of an examination which tested the person's ability to walk across a room. Those who could stagger, however slowly or painfully, across a confined space were denied the allowance. Yet, as Mrs R pointed out, 'When I was able to walk I could walk across a room but I couldn't get about outside.' Quite clearly the need for clear-cut administrative categories and a system that is easy to police denies help to many who are mobile only within the confines of their home. Secondly, many who were refused the allowance were angry because they knew of or had applied at the suggestion of others who received the benefit yet were more mobile than they. Mrs N was one of the most mobile persons among this group; she had a husband and daughters who owned cars and was able to walk to the local shops and back every day. She had been granted the allowance during an acute flare-up when she could not walk and continued to receive it despite her current abilities. Others lacking her physical capacities and personal resources got no help at all.

Some of the respondents felt that the welfare bureaucracy was unable to meet their needs because it was insufficiently flexible. As Mr M commented above, the rules and regulations governing eligibility were applied across the board, and there appeared to be no facility for taking into account special circumstances which rendered the rules inapplicable. Moreover, services and benefits when granted were not always delivered in a manner which suited the recipient but more often in a manner which suited the provider. Home helps might not come at the right time and might not be permitted to undertake tasks which were really needed. Benefits might be paid according to a timetable determined by the needs of the organization irrespective of the cash flow of the person receiving them and the inconveniences they might thereby experience. The cheque for Mr M's invalidity pension was issued on a Friday so did not arrive until Saturday or, if he was unlucky, the following Monday. Often this meant that he had little money to cover the weekend. His home help came on Friday, and one of her tasks was to buy sufficient food to enable him to manage Saturday and Sunday, and he never had enough money to pay her. Fortunately, she was prepared to use her own money to get the shopping, 'which I believe she shouldn't do officially', and he paid her back during the week when he had received his cheque. Without her co-operation, 'I would have had it, that's all there is to it.' He disliked having to rely on her kindness and disliked even more having to be in debt so asked if he might receive his cheque a day earlier: 'They said "No, your day is Friday." It's a rule, it's a rule, it's a rule and will not change. It's not designed to help you it's a convenience to them.' Over the year he too became increasingly bitter at having to struggle to obtain or being denied the resources he imagined were his right.

Conflict over definitions of need and how need was to be met was not confined to cash benefits but applied to other areas of provision. Differences of opinion existed over needs for telephones, housing, and aids and appliances, even the basic essentials of daily living, and a great deal of resentment was created when professionals and non-professionals acting on behalf of welfare agencies sought to impose their definitions on others. Mr M did not appreciate being told by social security officials that he should reduce his expenditure by getting rid of his television set; it was defined as a non-essential item even for someone living alone who was lucky to leave his flat once a week. The implication seemed to be that since he was out of work and subsisting on a limited income, he should not expect to have access to supposedly luxury items. Mr and Mrs I also greatly resented inquiries concerning their possessions. They stressed that they had worked hard in order to be able to buy a colour television set and freezer, both of which had been acquired and paid for before Mr I became disabled and unemployed. To them the implication seemed to be that if they were in possession of such supposedly luxury items, they could not be in need. Mrs A was not impressed by the response of the housing department when she turned down the offer of one local authority flat because it was too small for two people and badly affected by damp.

> *Mrs A:* We ended up having quite a fight, you know, they sort of shrugged their shoulders and said 'It's large enough for two' which we didn't believe and we just said 'No' and of course, we were told 'Well, then you'll just have to wait years.' In the end they were so unpleasant we got in touch with our MP.

The perception of the needs of disabled people entertained by some officials in this department were so inaccurate that they offered one of the respondents a flat on the fifth floor of a block, the living quarters of which could only be reached by going down seven narrow steps located just inside the front door. When Mrs W pointed out that she was confined to a wheelchair, the reply had been ' "Can't you get out of it while somebody carries it down for you?" '

Many of the respondents regarded themselves as, and indeed were, expert when it came to identifying their needs and the most efficient way of meeting them. They had lived with disability, knew their capabilities and limitations, and were well aware of the problems created by particular environments. Consequently, they were not too happy when occupational or rehabilitation therapists told them what was needed and did not allow them to decide for themselves. Mrs J had been supplied with aids and minor adaptations for the bathroom but found them relatively ineffective given her particular disabilities. She was unable to straighten her arms and could not reach the bath rails that had been positioned without regard for her limitations: 'This young lady came round and decided what I wanted and what I needed. Well, since they don't know me from Adam and never seen me in the bath I failed to see how they could decide what I want.' Again, some found it intolerable that they could not get the so-called experts to accept their definitions of need. Mrs R and her daughter had been trying for months to have their portable hoist serviced and weakened links in one of the chains repaired but without success. Their MP had telephoned on their behalf and still nothing was done.

> *Carol:* This is what I've found. If a piece of equipment goes wrong they won't believe you and this is so frustrating especially for a person like me because, OK, disabled people are used to being treated like imbeciles but I'm not disabled and the same attitude falls on me. They say 'But I can't understand what you mean,' and I say 'If you don't do something it will break,' and they say 'But I don't see how it can,' and they go on and on until it does break and they have proof. It's so frustrating 'cus we're the people using the equipment and we know when to look for danger signs and when we see them happening and nothing is done and our word isn't taken . . . you tend to think 'To hell with it,' no one's listening to me so I won't co-operate with them and this is when the disabled person suffers.

Conflicts over definitions of need or eligibility often developed into verbal conflicts between the respondents and the people who administered the system or otherwise provided help. In some cases it appeared that organizational representatives had to bear the brunt of the frustration created by the complexity and inequity of welfare provision; at other times it was generated by insensitivity or foolish remarks on their part. It was rare for Mrs I to emerge from her encounters with officers and clerks employed by the Department of Health and Social Security without feeling upset and angry. She found their attitude often left a great deal to be desired: 'They seem to put me down, you know what I mean? I know I'm down but I don't need them to tell me.' Mrs I was not alone in complaining of the treatment she received at the hands of some of those responsible for administering her case. Many had stories of off-hand comments that had been deeply hurtful and arguments created when moral judgements were handed out alongside or instead of much needed resources. Such encounters served only to heighten their sense of dependency at having to resort to welfare.

Mrs G: Everything you get you feel like a beggar, it's terrible. This woman came to see me to do something about clothing and I said 'I'd like some shoes 'cus they get out of shape, they get out of everything,' and she said 'If you're housebound you don't need any shoes.' I said 'Come on, I don't know what other people do but I don't slop around in slippers.' There again, it's like a rebuff you see, then you don't feel like going again which maybe is the idea, I don't know. You already feel awkward to ask for anything and then when you do they damned make a remark like that. You don't feel like going again.

Encounters between Mrs R and welfare organizations were often full of conflict, partly because she and her daughter were prepared to press their claims and partly because they had a great deal of experience of the insensitivity of representatives of those organizations and would no longer tolerate being treated with indifference. Mrs R said 'We've needed help so badly in the past when we haven't known people and we've rung the housing or the social services and got some cheeky girl and I've seen Carol in tears on the phone.' The most recent incident arose when she had asked if a home help could come more frequently for a short time to enable her daughter and son-in-law to go on holiday.

Mrs R: I had the most abusive telephone call, she was only a clerk that was working in home care and she said 'What's all this about them going on holiday?' So I said 'Well, what happens when they do go?' and she said 'Can't you even make yourself a cup of tea?' I said 'If you want me to put it crudely I can't wipe my bottom,' and it went off into a good old argument. She said, 'Well, you should go into a home.' Now honestly, to be spoken to like that!

Like Mrs G, Mrs R and her daughter interpreted such insensitivity as a deliberate strategy to head off claims for help. It was such a frequent occurrence that Carol always went prepared for a battle of wills: 'You have to be in a state of aggression ready to hit back at any remark they make.'

Even when the respondents had managed to establish their need and eligibility for a service or benefit, their problems were not at an end. Irrespective of the urgency of their need, it was rare that a benefit, service, or aid was supplied immediately; more likely the bureaucratic process involved meant delays of weeks if not months. In the meantime the persons concerned had to struggle on as best they could without the resources due to them. The last time Mrs R's hoist had broken it had been more than a month before it was repaired. Without the use of a hoist it was very difficult for her to get from her wheelchair to the bed and having a bath was out of the question. She was determined not to be put in that position again and enlisted the help of her MP, the manufacturer, and the law in order to have it serviced before it broke for a second time.

For those with financial problems, delays in getting benefits were particularly annoying. Soon after he moved into his adapted flat, Mr H applied for a mobility allowance, attendance allowance, and rent rebate, was examined and assessed for the first two and told he qualified for all three. Six months later he was still waiting, and in the meantime his rent and rates had increased substantially.

> *Mr H:* It's very distressing this income business. I applied months and months ago and I still haven't got a penny out of them. They keep saying it has to go through channels, so they say you'll get it in due course. And I say by the time I get anything I'll be dead. 'Oh, you'll get it in due course.' It's always in due course. I can't find out how much rent rebate I'll get and yet the rent's still got to be paid. Again it's, 'You'll hear in due course.' I'm fed up with keep phoning and asking and all they keep saying is they can't do anything about it it's going through the channels and it takes time.

At the first interview Mr M was very dispirited by the time it took to solve his problems, and he always seemed to be waiting for information, the answer to a question, a judgement concerning his entitlements to benefits, or an aid or appliance. Consequently, his personal circumstances seemed to improve very slowly.

> *Mr M:* Everything takes so long and I can never understand why it should. There seems to be no urgency about anything. It doesn't matter how the person who's waiting feels, this doesn't seem to count. I want to go back to work but you need help in that direction and I know if I go into that problem it's going to take months and months of waiting for the answer.

Because he was dependent upon a number of domiciliary services, his everyday existence was also characterized by waiting.

> *Mr M:* You've also got the problem that you're waiting for people to come in, the home help, people like that, you've got a lot of frustration waiting for people to come, home helps, meals on wheels. You're waiting for people all the time and you've got the added frustration if you have a bloody marvellous day and you feel you can go out that day it's, 'O Christ, I can't go, so and so's coming.' I look forward to the days I can be on my own. I know it sounds daft but I don't have to

worry about someone coming so I've got a little bit more freedom. But you're still lumbered 'cus the meals on wheels come. If you go anywhere you have to be back at such and such a time. Nothing is planned for what you want.

It was for this reason that Mrs W had done away with the formal home help service and now paid for domestic help. She had found herself 'a marvel' who was prepared to do anything and everything in the house, including walking the dog. She did not work fixed hours but stayed for however long it took her to complete her tasks. She was so trustworthy and efficient that Mrs W did not need to stay home to give her instructions and happily left the house in her care if she went away. This system was clearly far more satisfactory than the formal provision over which Mrs W had little control.

Occasionally the respondents would come across a provider who was able to circumvent the bureaucracy and solve their problems or supply their needs quickly. These individuals were highly regarded because they were effective and because they seemed to care. While delays were interpreted as indifference, efficient problem-solving was taken to indicate concern. Mr and Mrs I were very pleased with their rehabilitation officer who in the space of three weeks had managed to supply Mr I with the orthopaedic chair he requested and had given him a number of bathing aids. She was in the process of getting him a wheelchair to improve his mobility around the flat, was making enquiries about the possibility of his doing some work at home to relieve his boredom, and was planning a number of adaptations for when they were eventually rehoused. Summing up her contribution Mr I said 'She said it, she meant it, and she got 'em.' She was viewed as a useful ally in their struggle to improve their lot, and they were planning to ask for information about the mobility allowance at her next visit.

Nevertheless, such help, when it was found, sometimes appeared to be fragmented and discontinuous, attacking a small section of their problems rather than their problems as a whole. As Mr M said, 'They come in, solve a problem and then go away for a year. The lady that came today, I probably won't see her again', and the I's had not seen their rehabilitation officer since she had ordered a wheelchair for Mr I: 'I'd have thought she'd have popped in. I mean, she used to pop in twice a week. They just seem to come and then stay away.' The same applied to social workers. Those who said they did have a social worker found little continuity of care; their case seemed to be handed from one to the other without their knowledge so that, 'Everytime you ring up you get a different one.'

Housing was one resource for which the respondents expected and were prepared to wait but even here a great deal of distress was caused by uncertainty, a lack of information about the reasons for delay, and the apparent irrationality of the allocations systems. The majority of those still waiting to move were living in housing that was not only unsuitable for disabled people, but substandard and unsuitable for anyone. The blocks and streets in which they lived were being emptied prior to demolition or renovation. All had been given moving dates but these had passed with no offers of accommodation made, and they watched and waited as their able-bodied neighbours were given new housing and wondered why the disabled were not given priority. Mrs J gave up attempting to keep her eight-roomed house clean under the assumption that she was due to move, only to start again when the date she had been given passed. Mrs I began her packing assuming that the date she had been given would be honoured only to find this was not the case.

> *Mrs I:* Now they tell us it will be November. To me that's a lifetime. I built me hopes up and started packing and everything 'cus I thought we were moving and then they said 'about November'. It might not seem a long way off but when you're desperate it is.

The length of time it took for the local authority to rehouse its disabled tenants was probably explained by the nature of its housing stock; the units most readily available were not suited to the needs of disabled people, and it was necessary to wait until an adapted unit became vacant or was ready for occupation. If this was the case, then the respondents had not been informed. When they saw their neighbours rehoused, it seemed to them that they had been forgotten. Apart from receiving a letter giving her a moving date, Mrs J had heard nothing in the 18 months since she was assessed. Her attempts to locate the housing allocations officer had not met with success, and during the study year she had had to live with the uncertainty of not knowing what was happening in her case. Mr S had been so ill-informed that despite being severely disabled, he was not sure that he did qualify for an adapted or specially constructed accommodation and was unclear how to proceed to maximize his advantage. He was concerned that he might make the wrong decision and end up in another old flat or an area not to his liking.

> *Mr S:* That's the worry I've got now, will I be doing wrong taking a new flat or waiting for a disabled flat? The point is you wait for a disabled flat and you ain't going to get one, you don't know where you stand, you know. I think it should be one thing or another, they should notify you and let you know if you don't warrant a disabled flat or if you do. I must warrant a disabled flat. All right, you wait till you get one, but other than that you turn down all your good stuff. . . . They say you have three offers and the fourth one, don't matter where it is, you have got to take. I turn three good ones down here and they send me to China with the fourth where I don't want to go, you know, that's

the worry. If the first offer's a good flat I shall take the first offer because they haven't said I can have a disabled flat and they haven't said I can't. This way I know I'm going to get something decent.

Many of the respondents complained about the inefficiency of the welfare bureaucracy, particularly where it involved mistakes in the amount of benefits paid or the loss of application forms for services or other entitlements. Small matters loomed large simply because they seemed to typify the workings of the organizations on which the respondents were so dependent. Finding the solution to minor problems always seemed to involve a major exercise, with the respondents being passed from person to person and department to department until they could locate the one under whose jurisdiction the problem fell. Along the way they might be given different opinions concerning solutions to their problem or were sometimes told there was no provision for that particular problem and advised to pay for help themselves. In attempting to get the lead of his emergency bell extended so it would reach into the bedroom where he spent most of his time, Mr H tried the local housing department, the Social Services Department, the Greater London Council, and enlisted the help of his rehabilitation officer but was told by all that they were not authorized to do it, and it would have to be done privately. Two weeks after he paid for the lead to be extended an electrician turned up at his flat with an order to do the job for him. Similarly, when he moved into the flat he was told that as a severely disabled person, he was able to get financial help with a telephone; after he had paid for it to be installed he was told that he was not entitled to help as he had a bell which he could use to summon help in an emergency. While these sorts of problems are an additional source of irritation disabled people can well do without, it is their implication that is more important. As Mr H said, 'This is the kind of bureaucratic muddle we live in, the right hand doesn't know what the left hand is doing . . . nobody seems to give a damn.' At the end of a discussion of his difficulty of mobilizing formal help, Mr M said 'I get the impression they don't know what they're doing. I'm not sure they know themselves. They all ask the same questions.'

Coping with the welfare bureaucracy

The skills and resources needed to manage the problems created by the welfare bureaucracy were not evenly distributed among the respondents. Some of those who were experiencing or had experienced problems were conspicuously more adept at getting providers to respond to their needs. They possessed the knowledge and the social skills necessary for pursuing their claims and could often mobilize others to put pressure on organizations responsible for services or benefits. Perhaps the most fundamental asset in this respect is knowledge of the system and how it operates and knowledge of the critertia determining eligibility for welfare. Knowledge was not only useful for constructing the most advantageous package of services and benefits but also useful during conflicts with the experts. Probably the best informed among this group of people were Mrs R and her daughter, who knew their rights and would go to whatever lengths necessary to pursue them. They frequently gave advice and information to other disabled people and would also assist them with campaigns in support of their claims. Consequently, their relationship with the local Social Services Department was an unhappy one.

> *Carol:* It's a case of knowing too much. We know the rules, we know the regulations, we know the Chronically Sick and Disabled Persons Act and if you're having a barny with a senior social worker and they give you a load of drivel and you turn round and say 'No, because under section whatever of the Act', it's 'Well we don't want to have anything to do with you, you know too much.'
> *Mrs R:* I think this is rather unfair. On the one hand we're told to do all we can for ourselves but on the other if you do go against the authorities and stand up for yourself you're immediately put down as a rebel. I'm the biggest rebel around, I'm certain of that.

Not all the respondents were as knowledgeable as this and often found their attempts to clarify their own position with respect to entitlements frustrated. One problem was that the rules and regulations governing provision were framed in a language that was not readily accessible to the uninitiated. Mr M said 'one wants the information what one is entitled to', and then pointed to a number of official leaflets he had received which made detailed reference to a number of acts of Parliament: 'Now the average lay person has no chance of finding out what this lot means.' In addition, the structure of the bureaucracy and the distribution of responsibility is so complex that it is difficult to identify and locate an individual who can give comprehensive information and advice about rights and entitlements. The fragmentation of the service prevents easy access of such information.

> *Mr I:* It spreads over so many different departments. The rehab lady might come down and we ask her about school meals and she said 'That's not my department, I don't know about that.' You want somebody who knows about the lot.
> *Mrs I:* All of 'em, so you know what forms and what you're filling in. There's one care allowance, one invalid allowance, one mobility allowance, well apparently it's all different departments.
> *Mr I:* With the kiddies' clothing grants and school meals you speak to

someone and 'I don't know anything about it. It's not my department.'
They can only help you in their own department.
Mrs I: You want someone who knows the lot, where to go and how to
do it. There must be someone like that, someone who floats about and
knows everything, like, you know.

Mr M had also experienced difficulty learning about what was
available, and until he discovered a booklet listing locally available
services, he had to rely on others. Once having found out that he was
eligible for a free holiday, he was able to telephone the Social Services and
arrange one for himself without the intervention of an intermediary: 'It all
goes back to information you see.'

Mr and Mrs I not only found it difficult to obtain the information they
required, they also had trouble in giving the necessary information to
support their claims. The application forms they had been given proved a
major problem, and they had not been able to obtain help in filling them
in correctly. They wondered whether they might have been refused
benefits simply because they had misunderstood the forms and not given
the correct information. Mrs I said 'I put down husband's wages and
wife's wages but all them other questions I'm lost 'cus I've never had to do
it before.' In the context of limited social skills, other procedures involved
in the bureaucratic process were equally problematic. Mrs I had been
called to an Appeals Tribunal in the course of their claim for an invalid
care allowance and found the experience so harrowing that she was
reluctant to press their claim for help with a telephone in case it led to
another similar hearing.

> *Mrs I:* I was frightened again about getting in front of another one.
> Next time I'll take somebody a bit more . . . 'cus they use great big long
> words, you know. When I went last time I was saying 'Pardon? What?'
> I said 'I'm sorry, I just don't understand your way of speaking,' I said
> ' 'cus it doesn't mean anything to me, you've got to bring it down to my
> level' I said.

The I's were among the sub-group of people who did not have the
personal contacts of the kind which can be useful in short-cutting the
bureaucratic process or otherwise affecting the outcome of their claims.
Since their social worker had withdrawn, they had had no formal or
informal support in their attempt to secure their entitlements and better
their lot. They were unaware of the existence of organizations that
assisted disabled people to get services and benefits and had only recently
become aware of the Citizens Advice Bureau as a source of help. Other
respondents had personal contacts who worked in the bureaucracy, or
were known to members of the borough council or their MP, and used
them to exert pressure on organizations which were slow to respond or

otherwise treated them in ways they considered unfair. At one time Mrs R had contacts in the office of the Minister for the Disabled and often called on them to help in her battles with the Social Services Department. When living in appalling housing conditions, she used her contacts and appeared on a local television programme and soon after was rehoused by the local authority's housing department. When Mrs W was threatened with eviction from her council flat because she contravened regulations by keeping a dog, she spoke to a number of councillors she knew, who intervened on her behalf, and was allowed to keep both the dog and the flat. On occasions even influential others were unsuccessful in getting the bureaucracy to move and a more militant strategy had to be adopted.

> *Mrs R:* We kept on and on 'Would they come and see to the hoist?' because the chain was coming apart and they should be serviced every three years. They completely ignored us and in the end I got X to ring from the Minister's office and it was still ignored and nothing was done so we threatened to take out a court order and then they started moving. Yesterday Carol was getting me from the chair to bed and it broke. Luckily I was over the bed at the time, but this is the sort of thing they can't afford to let happen.
> *Carol:* Two months ago I got so desperate I rang the manufacturers thinking it was their hoist and they were very concerned they said 'Get a new chain fitted' but they didn't have the manpower to come. Well, when I rang Social Services they said 'You had no right to go to the manufacturers without our knowledge,' but I said 'It's dangerous. Something was going to happen.' I said 'I've been ringing you, the Minister's office have been ringing you and you've taken no notice. What are we supposed to do?' and it was still 'You had no right to go to the manufacturers.' And because we went over their heads their way of getting back, well, 'We won't do it.' And as soon as the court action was threatened they were going to do it, actually today, but then the hoist broke on Monday and whereas before they said it couldn't be done immediately they came immediately.

For Mrs R, the problem she experienced in getting her hoist repaired was not unusual but fairly typical of the welfare bureaucracy and its response to requests for help. Without the kind of pressure she was able to exert, help only became available at times of crisis, usually when it was too late. She was able to present numerous case histories from among her extensive network of disabled people where tragedies had been allowed to happen because help had not been given at the right time. She could only speculate as to what might have happened had she not been fortunate enough to be suspended over the bed when her hoist broke. Whatever the validity of her view of the welfare bureaucracy, and there is support for it in the literature (Stevenson and Parsloe 1978), it explained her own militancy when dealing with agencies charged with the welfare of disabled people. While her militant and aggressive approach had initially been adopted as a result of despair, it was now adopted because it had proved to be the only effective approach. For example, when she moved into her current accommodation, she discovered her hoist needed some minor modifications to allow her to use it for getting into and out of the bath. She was told by the Social Services Department that it would take at least nine months to have it altered and she was not prepared to wait that long because bathing was the most efficient way of keeping clean and one way of securing some relief from pain: 'I don't know what made me do it but I rang them back and said "If you don't do anything about the hoist it's no good to me and it's going in the road." They still wouldn't do anything about it so we put it in the road.' Mrs R called a reporter from the local press; the story and a photograph appeared in the paper the following Friday, and by Wednesday she was taking a bath. There was only one conclusion to be drawn from these experiences: 'You see they *can* do it but you've got to fight for it to be done. It just needs a little bit of a push, they can do it with a little bit of pressure.' Nevertheless, she did add 'It wears you out, this fighting that the disabled have to do, it's so bad, we shouldn't have to fight.'

Not all the respondents were prepared to go to the same lengths as Mrs R but did try to speed up the process by making repeated phone calls to the organizations concerned. This strategy was not always successful, and there was a limit to how far the people concerned were prepared to pursue those dealing with the case. After four months of telephoning and waiting for a rehabilitation officer to call, Mrs A enlisted the help of a local councillor and was finally visited, only to discover that she now had to wait months for the borough surveyor to call to give an opinion on the adaptations that had been recommended: 'I don't feel inclined to keep bothering them and I really don't know what to do.' Mr M had tried this strategy only to find that, 'If you chase these people up they don't like it, at least this is my impression, you get the impression from them you're nothing but a ruddy inconvenience,' and Mrs T felt she was less effective in pressuring others than she might be: 'I sometimes wish I had a slightly different temperament and couldn't always see someone else's point of view, you know, just see my goal and not think about anyone else.' Without the capacity or the inclination to force the issue, there was nothing to it but to wait.

The process of acquiring benefits and services was often long and arduous and might involve convoluted arguments about eligibility and rates of pay. Mr S and Mrs K had been subjected to months of argument and counter-argument before they were granted the attendance allowance and the system began to run smoothly, and Mrs D had been waiting for nine months for her appeal for a mobility allowance to be heard. The irritation generated was very much resented by people who had better things to do with their energy. Even Mr H, who took the same attitude towards the bureaucracy as Mrs R and who, now confined to bed, spent his time 'putting rockets under people' he considered less than efficient, was dispirited by the process. His whole time seemed to be spent dealing with organizations and officials who provided for his needs.

> *Mr H:* But quite honestly when you're ill for long you get sick of argy-bargy with people, arguing with people about rent and rate rebates, are you getting the attendance allowance? Are you getting the mobility allowance? The central heating things, they've packed up and didn't work at all. What a terrible job we had getting them fixed, it went on for weeks and weeks. You get sick of this argy-bargy, and everything. You've got to send them letters. Send them a letter, you just keep sending letters *all* the time.

The effort involved in dealing with the bureaucracy can become so great that the individual simply gives up and withdraws and ceases to press his or her claims or apply for further entitlements. Mrs G had been caught up in a long legal dispute with a former employer over an administrative error which had cost her a great deal in lost sick pay. Although she had a good case she had now let it drop: 'They tell me to go on but I'm too tired, I like peace of mind now, I like peace.' On a more mundane level she had been caught in the middle of a dispute over a clothing allowance, and although they did eventually give her a grant for a coat and a dress, she declined the offer of further provision and though now eligible for additional help had decided not to reapply. Withdrawal from the system did not always follow disputes, arguments, or lengthy administrative procedures. A simple refusal of a claim sometimes caused such bitterness that no further claims were made. This was particularly the case where an examination was off-hand or cursory and no explanation given to justify ineligibility. Mr F had applied for a mobility allowance on the recommendation of a friend and could not understand why he had been turned down. The doctor undertaking the assessment had not given him a proper examination, merely asked him a few questions, and Mr F could only surmise that it was because he had been self-employed, and they assumed he was 'rotten with money'.

> *Mr F:* I did think about applying for that again and help with the road tax but I don't think I shall bother. I don't know how to put it . . . when the doctor turned round and told me I couldn't have it it upset me quite a lot. Probably I had no right to be there in the first place but it did upset me. When I came home I said, 'That's it', I just wouldn't bother again. I

just wouldn't lower myself to go back because if he was there again then that would upset me a damn sight worse and I'd be liable to say something stupid so I haven't bothered to reapply.

Given the difficulties many had experienced in their dealings with agents and agencies charged with promoting their welfare, many perceived the system as one hostile to them and their needs; they were left feeling abandoned by an institution that was created to care. This was a frightening prospect for those who did not have alternative sources of social and economic support. As Mrs R said, 'If they won't help you who do you turn to?' It is, perhaps, not surprising that those who had such resources were noticeably less critical of welfare provision than those without.

A crisis in the family

As I mentioned in the previous chapter, Mrs R was very troubled by what she regarded as a significant gap in welfare provision, the absence of immediate help to assist in containing conflict in the home. She returned to this topic a number of times during the interviews and following arguments with her daughter had tried to locate an individual or an organization who would be available at short notice but was without success.

> *Mrs R:* What happens when something goes wrong in the home which it does in every home but especially with a disabled person 'cus we are difficult, there's no doubt about it. I get annoyed because there's no one you can contact and it frightens me because this is the time we've known tragedies to happen. Social Services you can never contact at weekends so where do you go?

Mrs R's concern proved to be well founded. A few months after the second interview an argument in her family developed into a major conflict, leading to a temporary breakdown in her relationship with her daughter and her admission to residential care. In this case help was available, both formal and informal, but it proved to be the wrong kind of help at the wrong time. Her account of the argument and its aftermath are presented as an illustration of the way in which intervention by friends and welfare agencies, coupled with poor communication and misunderstanding of the needs of the people concerned, can damage rather than promote their interests. The story also raises more fundamental questions about power and responsibility: professional intervention can mean a loss of control so that the client has things done to them rather than for them. The account is not offered as an example of what typically happens, although Mrs R and her daughter came to view it in that way, but as an illustration of how easily situations can develop a momentum of their own and end, almost, in tragedy. The rift in the family had begun as a domestic argument which, given its immediate context, had taken on a more significant character.

Mrs R: It was purely through an ordinary domestic upset that had been building up and building up and if we'd had some co-operation and some help it would never have happened. Everytime I wanted anything done like my hoist or my bed seeing to it was, well, 'Can't Carol use a screwdriver? Can't she do it' and this had been building up. I had a lot of resentment against her husband and he's bought some property and was trying to get started in business and this was another drag on them and it all blew up out of proportion. It was one of those situations which build up suddenly whereas if it had been left it would have been all right. When we quarrel it isn't particularly nice and that night if they had gone out and left me for an hour or two which they didn't or if I could have got into my car and driven it around for an hour which I couldn't. If I could have spoken to someone who understood and we could have aired our differences it wouldn't have come to anything, but you see, I was getting so annoyed and so upset and in the end I rang the one person who was the last person I should have rung. She couldn't get round quick enough and instead of saying 'this is silly' she turned completely on Carol and I was upset and probably said a lot of things I shouldn't, I think I said I didn't want to see them ever again.

Carol and her husband left, and Mrs R ended up so distressed that her friend contacted Social Services, and she was immediately taken into a home.

Mrs R: It was a most awful place, you felt as if you were waiting to die. I swear if I'd been there a week I wouldn't have been here, I'd have gone completely . . . I never spoke to anyone that first day. The staff were very good but the people there were all very confused. They just sat around waiting. I don't know what they were waiting for. Do you know, they even encourage you to be incontinent. I couldn't believe it. I was put in the sick bay and the first night the matron came in and said someone will look in every hour but on the second night I was absolutely horror stricken she came in and said 'There are only two people on duty tonight so if you want to go to the toilet we've got a special thing on the bed, don't be afraid just go.' Then they wouldn't let me out. It was a nightmare. They said 'No, we can't let you go, you can't do anything for yourself.' I said 'You haven't given me a chance to try, I've got to prove I can do something for myself,' but they refused to let me out. It was a nasty frightening thing.

Int: How did you manage to get out?

Mrs R: Only through my doctor coming. After my doctor and the consultant came the matron came in and said 'Your doctors have backed you up, we can't keep you,' and the whole atmosphere changed. I think they were treating me as if I was stupid because after all this they were saying 'You're a very intelligent person.' They wanted me to stay in the home over the weekened but I just couldn't, I insisted on coming home.

Mrs R was brought home in an ambulance accompanied by three social workers, and soon after, Carol and her husband arrived to see if she was all right.

Carol: I still can't believe it happened. Mum was completely surrounded by these three social workers and I wasn't able to get to her, you know, they interfered every time I sort of went to say 'Mum, are you all right?' 'Yes she is.' You know, they were answering for her. Jack was absolutely horrified and didn't know what to do and he said 'Well, I'm not leaving' and the social workers said 'You've got to go' and he said 'I'm not leaving my mother like this.' 'Well,' they said 'we'll get the police to evict you', which they did. And the policeman didn't know what was going on. He said 'The best thing you can do is just go and leave it to them and when they've messed it up it'll be your turn to come back.' I kept saying to them 'I want to be sure my mother will be attended to if I do go' and in front of the police officer they said 'We can assure you we will make sure she's all right.' What we didn't know was that as soon as we'd left they'd left. There again, they refused to give me any information. I didn't know mum had been taken to a home, if I'd known I'd have gone straight away and said you're coming out, I'd just come to see if she was all right and cleverly they locked the doors so I couldn't get in. I said to the policeman 'Can you make them give me information if she drops dead? Are you going to inform me?' They said 'We have no legal obligation to notify you of anything.' So I thought 'To hell with you, to hell with everything, if you're going to take that attitude.' And I said 'You're all here now, where were you when we needed help months ago, where were you then?' I just can't explain, I've never felt so humiliated, I'll never forget that humiliation. So I said, 'To hell with it I'm not putting up with this, if these people want to take over, let them and good luck to them.'

Soon after Carol and her husband left, the social workers left too and Mrs R had to begin to cope alone.

Mrs R: The only thing they did I got one of them to undo the zip of my dress. They just left me. I had nothing. My bed was higher than my wheelchair, my chair had no brakes, I had no helping hand, I had nothing, it was a nightmare. I think I managed to get to bed about four in the morning, the sweat was pouring off me, you can't imagine the effort. The place was a bit of a mess, I couldn't get to the toilet, I was drinking milk out of a pint bottle of milk. Carol's been looking after me for nine years and to be suddenly put back . . . to be suddenly dumped back after getting all this attention and completely left. I was absolutely without help for that first night, it was the longest night of my life. The next morning I had a tummy upset and I managed to get from the bed to the chair a couple of times in the morning and I tried to do it again and of course as I went to get into the chair it moved away 'cus it didn't have any brakes and I went on the floor. The least the social workers could have done was to make sure my chair was safe. Anyway I didn't know what to do and the phone kept ringing and I managed to get to that. It was the manager from the housing department and all I was frightened of was they'd send me back to the home if they heard I had a fall. They're going to say you can't manage and send me back so erm I said 'Look, I'm not hurt and everyone has a fall at some times, can you get someone to get me up?' As I say I did manage to keep going for about five weeks. The district nurses were absolutely marvellous and I had meals on wheels. The nurses came in the morning and again in the afternoon and put me to bed so that meant I was in bed at four o'clock and wouldn't see anyone till the following morning. I used to panic though, I used to think 'Are the doors locked? Have I got my Helping Hand? Have I got a drink?' And I used to worry 'cus I used to think if anything gets moved what am I going to do. I mean I would have got used to all that. I'm glad I didn't have to.

During her five weeks of coping without her daughter, Mrs R felt pressured by the housing department, who seemed to want her to give up the house.

Mrs R: They were trying so hard to get me out of here, this is what annoys me so much. One night the housing manager came, he just walked in, I wasn't feeling very happy and he said 'Oh no, you can't stay here.' Now I was so taken aback, I said 'What do you mean?' He said 'You can't stay here, you can't do this, you can't do that.' But I said 'You haven't given me a chance, I want my bed lowered, I want a ring so I can make a cup of tea.' I saw him the other day and I was so annoyed over it. He said 'If you want the truth I was told by Social Services you were going into Part III accommodation permanently.'
Int: You say you went into hospial for a week?
Mrs R: I'm a bit ashamed to say . . . I'll tell you what happened. Now, I've never missed paying my rent, I pay it every month by cheque but what I didn't know, Carol told me afterwards, that had been changed and had to be paid weekly. Instead of telling me this, they knew very

well I was on my own, the next thing a letter arrived stating that if the arrears weren't paid I'd be evicted. All this doing was going on, apart from the fact that I missed Carol so much, all these things were happening, don't ask me why, I can't explain why but I'd had this one friend coming and she'd taken over completely. She used the phone, she used the bath, and she said one day 'I was thinking of taking your car, I'm having driving lessons and it'll save me getting one of my own' and I think this pulled me up 'cus I live to drive and she went one Sunday evening and was coming back the next morning and honestly, I couldn't face it. I rang my doctor, now if I could have spoken to him nothing would have happened but my doctor was on holiday, well, I don't know, I just took more tablets that I should. I did ring my brother and tell him and he got an ambulance. But you know, it frightens me how quickly it can happen. It's not that I thought 'I'm sick of living I want to do this, I want to get out.' But it scared me how easily that thing can happen, I didn't feel a thing.

During the weeks they were apart, no one attempted to mediate between Mrs R and Carol, and neither realized that the other was unhappy at the separation. Mrs R thought that Carol would not want to come back once she had tasted freedom and felt it was best for her to have a life of her own, and Carol imagined she had been smothering her mother and was not wanted back: 'There wasn't a single person who tried to get us together or said "Let's talk." They seemed to be pushing us down all the time.' A reconciliation occurred soon after Mrs R came home from hospital and was forced to phone Carol because the district nurse had refused to give her an injection when she needed one because of pain.

Mrs R: It was only then that we realized that none of us could have stood it that way. We're all so grateful to be back because it's cleared the air 'cus I had a lot of resentment against Jack which was eating away into me but that's gone now, that's all finished. At least they came back of their own accord. I hated every minute of it, I don't mind saying that now.

Clearly, primary prevention had not been successful in this case, and for whatever reason help had only become available when it was too late, when the problem had reached crisis point and resource input had to be that much greater. In the context of scarce resources, it is not unreasonable for services to be directed at those most in need, in this case disabled people living alone with no one on whom they can rely. Nevertheless, numerous research reports have shown that families caring for a disabled or elderly person do need some support so that the considerable costs of community care are not wholly borne by the family. The needs of Mrs R and Carol were not considerable; they would have been contented with some formal recognition of Carol's caring role and the payment of a benefit sufficient to compensate for loss of occupational and other opportunities. They would also have appreciated having an uninvolved party to call on who could assist at the few times when the strain of caring and the strain of being a burden became too much. They would have settled for prompt attention when a piece of equipment essential in helping them cope with the daily grind required repair. And having reached crisis point they would have liked formal or informal support that was more sensitive to their needs.

Looking back on the incident and its consequences, Mrs R was quite clear about the extent to which intervention fuelled and prolonged the crisis when all that was needed was a little sympathetic counselling.

> *Mrs R:* It was one of those situations that had it been left it would have been all right. After the argument happened if it had been left as it was everything would have returned to normal. This is another thing that's worried me a great deal because I never really believed it when I used to hear people say 'Oh no, I wouldn't contact Social Services, they only make things worse.' I used to think 'That's stupid, don't be silly.' Now, I would never contact them in that kind of a situation again because it's taken completely out of your hands. All we needed was someone to say 'This is ridiculous, you and Carol have never been apart.' I get the impression they didn't want us to be united in any way. It nearly destroyed us.

For whatever reason, the decisions made on Mrs R's behalf did not seem to facilitate or promote independent living but appeared to be leading her into a greater dependence on formal care. The informal assistance she received while living alone appeared to be equally disabling. It was only through her own determination that she was given the chance to develop the skills to cope without the degree of personal care to which she had become accustomed. The formal support she received during this transition period was not supportive and even the nursing care, while highly valued, was organized so that it often left her trapped in bed at four in the afternoon. Presumably, a better arrangement would have evolved over time as Mrs R learned to cope with living alone. In the event, that proved not to be necessary as family relationships were restored, cleansed of the tension that helped promote the initial rift. The incident then became the latest in a long series of struggles that had been characteristic of her life. Looking back over her career as a disabled person, Mrs R echoed many of the respondents' experiences. She said 'I've been through so much in my life, you know, so many things. I've been through the war, I've worked, I've brought up children. People have said to me "Well, I just don't know how you can get through those things." But I've managed to. I've had to fight all of my life. Ever since I can remember, I've had to fight.'

Conclusion

In describing the experiences of twenty-four men and women severely disabled by rheumatoid arthritis, an attempt has been made to convey something of the impact of chronic illness on everyday life in particular and life chances in general. In the context of chronic illness even the mundane activities of daily life can no longer be taken for granted. The simplest tasks become a problem, of sometimes gargantuan proportions, so that time and other resources may be wholly absorbed in attempting to accomplish them in satisfactory ways. Chapters 2 to 7 have attempted to describe in some detail the problems that this group of people encountered, the strategies they employed in order to solve or manage these problems, and the resources that were available to help them. In giving descriptions of their everyday affairs, the people who took part in the study were able to demonstrate the suffering, distress, and frustration created by a chronic disabling illness and to illustrate the poverty of an existence characterized by pain, loss of physical capacity, and the never-ending effort of coping with day-to-day living. It is hoped that something of this remains in the extracts and analysis presented.

While essentially a detailed description of one chronic illness and its consequences, the study was also intended to address a number of theoretical concerns. These were largely derived from Wood's model of impairment, disability, and handicap and the variable sequence of events which may link physical loss or malfunction and social disadvantage. That is, the resources people command and the strategies they employ to solve their problems are factors which modify the impact of impairment and disability and moderate disadvantage in everyday life. The empirical approach was derived from the previous work of sociologists broadly identified as interactionists, predominantly Strauss and his colleagues. In this way the study had the somewhat ambitious aim of contributing to two radically different traditions. In focusing on the multiple problems encountered by a small group of people limited by one chronic disorder, it was intended to say something about the nature and character of handicap and to illustrate the idea that the meaning of impairment and disability is influenced by social and environmental contexts. At the same time it has tried to verify and elaborate some of the issues and themes addressed by writers such as Wiener, Strauss, and Reif and the more recent contributions of Shearer and Bury.

Some of the problems described in preceding chapters may appear familiar to people who are not impaired or disabled in any way. It is certainly not the case that the lives of the healthy are always harmonious and trouble free, even if they are employed, have adequate incomes, decent housing, and active social lives. The lives of disabled people are different if only because of the sheer volume of problems they face and their cumulative effects. People with disorders like rheumatoid arthritis carry a double burden; the symptoms of the disease can be so devastating that the physical or psychological resources needed to cope with the broader personal and social consequences of disability are simply not available. It is for this reason that medical care occupies such an important place in the lives of many chronically sick people. Despite being aware of its limitations, the respondents in this study continued to look to medical science for ways of minimizing pain and restoring damaged joints. Medicine has other important functions which go beyond mere therapeutic intervention. It is a source of knowledge and, though incomplete, provides an explanatory framework which facilitates the search for meaning in experience. It is also a source of hope; whatever their views of the efficacy of the care they had received, many respondents continued to believe that medical science would come up with a cure or a drug to control their pain. They also looked to medicine and its practitioners for social and psychological support and, arguably, this was its most significant contribution. If the chronically sick and disabled person had no place and no status in the wider society, he or she did have a place within the context of medical care; hence their distress when they came to believe that they were no longer valued by the doctors dealing with their case, when they felt written off by society at large and its caring institutions. It appeared that much was to be gained when doctors maintained an interest in their clinical condition and their personal and social affairs, if only because they felt valued as a result. Like those interviewed by Bury (1982), the people in this study evidenced no wholesale rejection of medicine despite their understanding of its current limitations and their sometimes severe criticisms of those involved in practice. As the data in Chapter 2 has demonstrated, some of the respondents experienced difficulties in their relationships with doctors so that many of the potential benefits of medical practice went unclaimed.

Coping with a disease like rheumatoid arthritis highlights the crucial role of knowledge in chronic illness. It is a powerful resource, facilitating the practical management of the disorder and the emotional adaptation to the illness and its effects. This explains the irritation of some of the respondents who believed their doctors were withholding information necessary for coping with arthritis and its future implications. A comparison of the concerns voiced by Bury's respondents and those interviewed here suggests that the need for knowledge varies during the course of the illness career. In the initial stages there is a concern with the problem of onset, with finding an answer to the question of why they have acquired a disease usually considered a complaint of the elderly. Although nearly all are told that no cause is known, they arrive at causal explanations by reinterpreting doctors' comments and questions, by invoking commonsense connections between stressful events and illness, and by searching personal and family biographies in order to give some coherence to the whole. In the later stages of the career, they come face to face with a different kind of uncertainty. The significance of the problem of onset declines as they become overwhelmed by the need to account for the day-to-day variation in levels of pain and activity and the need to have a clear idea of their prognosis. These are essential for managing the disorder, both in the short and the long term. Because medicine cannot provide satisfactory answers to these questions, they are left to impose certainty on uncertainty in whatever way they can.

Chronic illness leading to a loss of physical capacity immediately calls into question the resources an individual has to hand. What may have been adequate prior to disability are rendered inadequate to compensate for physical loss and provide for a satisfactory existence within the community. The problem of resources becomes more acute over time as emerging disability sees the erosion of income, wealth and, in some cases, social support. Disabled people face the problem of managing their illness and its effects with resources which do not match those they enjoyed when able bodied.

When people no longer have the strength or manual dexterity to perform everyday tasks or where they are virtually immobilized by pain, the nature and extent of the resources they continue to command have a significant effect on life chances. Available resources will determine whether a valued activity can be maintained or has to be abandoned, or in the case of essential activities like personal care or household management, a wide range of resources may allow individuals to choose from among a number of possible solutions to their problems. They may decide to pay for help themselves, they may prefer to have help from family or friends, or they may decide to seek help from voluntary or statutory bodies. Or they may decide to try each of the options in turn, until one is found to more nearly meet their needs or to give rise to few additional problems. Money is a significant resource in this respect. Buying help on the open market may be preferable to the help given by a formal service because the buyer retains control over what is provided and can choose to employ whosoever is willing to offer the kind of help they want. It makes it easier to acquire the right kind of help at the right time and does not compromise their independence. Those who do not have the means to buy help must put up with formal services which operate according to their own timetables and provide the help they think is needed, or must call on relatives and friends and tolerate feeling and being a burden on others. In this respect the debate concerning the merits of benefits in cash and benefits in kind is of continuing relevance. Benefits in kind create dependency and limit choice; benefits in cash may have their own defects but allow disabled people to retain the self determination and dignity taken for granted by their non-disabled counterparts (Shearer 1981a). While disabled people have similar problems, their individual needs can be highly idiosyncratic. It is probably beyond the bounds of human ingenuity to design a formal service which is ideal from the perspectives of providers and individual consumers. Benefits in cash allow the recipients to design their own and thereby avoid the problems many of them experience during their contacts with a professional service.

Clearly, the meaning of a given disability is not the same to all who are limited in similar ways. The problems that arise from a given activity restriction may be more or less manageable according to the resources that are available. Knowledge, money, aids and appliances, and adapted environments may lead to independence in daily living and access to wider opportunities. Among the group of people interviewed, there were significant differences in the types and amounts of resources they had in hand. Some received financial support adequate to meet their basic living expenses while others did not, some had extensive social networks on whom they could call while others were isolated, and some lived in housing more suited to their needs while some had to tolerate domestic environments that disabled rather than enabled. There were also conspicuous differences in knowledge and social skills so that some were more adept in their dealings with the providers of medical and social care. Bury (1982) has suggested that such resources are variably distributed in society, that individuals from some social strata are less able to manage the effects of disability and reduce the hardship it produces, at least in the long term. A study based on a small group of people is an inadequate basis from which to generalize and cannot be used to support or challenge that point of view. Data from these case studies does, however, tend to suggest a complex picture so that hardship and unhappiness are not exclusively the lot of individuals drawn from the lower socio-economic groups. Opportunities for remaining in work following the onset of disability were not markedly different for those employed in manual and non-manual occupations, and the presence of supportive social networks were not confined to individuals of one particular social class. Similarly, the location of activities which offered an acceptable alternative to work seemed to be influenced more by sex than previous occupation. If anything, there was more evidence to support Shearer's (1981a) sugges- tion that the greater resources were commanded by and directed towards those least in need. The philosophy of 'rewarding the able-bodied' implicit in welfare provision did seem to bias the services in favour of the relatively strong.

Such questions are, of course, only properly addressed by studies using larger and randomly selected samples which employ some measure of handicap in order to facilitate comparisons between groups. While we now have sophisticated measures of impairment and disability which provide the opportunity to undertake research aimed at identifying factors involved in the onset and development of impairment and disability, there is no such measure of disadvantage or handicap. Wood (1980) has offered a classification of handicaps but this is in no way a measure. Handicap is currently vaguely defined and consequently difficult to operationalize, and until we have an adequate instrument it is necessary to work with indicators such as income, rates of unemployment, and social isolation which address an important part, but by no means the whole, of the problem. While we have gone a long way towards the development of techniques which allow us to study the natural history of impairment and disability, we have yet to develop a technology for assigning a numerical value to their consequences in everyday life. The techniques employed by Brown and Harris (1979) in their studies of the social origins of depression have indicated ways in which we might begin to measure meaning. All that it is safe to say on the basis of the present data is that all the respondents required additional resources of some kind, though their individual needs varied widely.

These comments apply not only to occupation and social class and their relationship to resources, coping abilities, and the social consequences of chronic illness, but to all the factors and processes which may intervene between impairment, disability, and handicap. The emphasis on this study has been on social resources and social coping and has said little of psychological processes and their role in the sequence of events outlined by Wood (1980). Nor has the study been able to demonstrate, since it did not intend to do so, differences in long-term life chances between people who had access to different amounts or types of resources. Such an enterprise requires a detailed understanding of the nature of handicap, a method of measuring social disadvantage in all its forms, a theoretical appreciation of the dynamics of handicap, and studies with relatively sophisticated research designs. Only then will it be possible to identify key variables and the part they play in the development of handicap and only then will it be possible to create interventions, at least at the individual level, to help disabled people limit the consequences of a given disorder.

While research of that kind would allow for the identification of key resources and coping mechanisms which can be supplemented and enhanced as part of the process of securing the integration of the disabled individual in community life, enough has been written about the barriers to integration and the wider social origins of disadvantage and deprivation to enable more effective policy options to be identified. Some of these call for an expansion in current provision, some call for a reform of provision to remove inequality of treatment between disabled people with equivalent needs, and some call for a fundamentally different kind of provision. All of these discussions identify a set of basic needs; those of physical access to the community, improved mobility, an income that does more than just cover the bare necessities of daily living, some kind of work or meaningful way of occupying time, and independent living with the help of suitable domestic environments and domiciliary support which facilitates that goal. It is difficult to choose among these needs to identify one which is of overriding importance; in part, because they are not discrete but overlap and, in part, because the fulfilment of one facilitates the fulfilment of the others. Other important needs would include access to information to enable them to manage their condition and easier access to services designed to help. As it is, seeking help may increase the burden disabled people experience as a result of their disorder and its effects in everyday life.

In order to improve the lot of disabled people, some have called for a shift in resources to make effective community care a reality (Townsend 1981) and some for a comprehensive disability income based on need and not the place or circumstance of onset (Walker 1981). The challenge, however, is not only to provide services to meet these needs but to provide them in a manner which does not create dependency and a devalued status. We have long recognized that institutional care, while able to provide for some of the basic requirements of the long-term sick and disabled population, dehumanizes and depersonalizes by making the individual subordinate to a regime which meets the needs of the organization but not the individual. The same critical eye could be directed with equal benefit to the way we help those who live in the community. This help may also limit independence and constrain choice. Some experimental schemes have demonstrated that care can be provided in a manner which suits the particular needs of the individual, thereby allowing even severely disabled people to stay in their own homes (Bristow 1981). Given the complexity and fragmentation of the services which exist for disabled people, there also appears to be a need for a specially trained worker to give advice about benefits and services and also to act as an advocate during their attempts to construct the most favourable package out of what is available (Glendinning 1981).

There are, of course, constraints on the nature and volume of services offered to the disabled population which go beyond those of cost. Social values are of some significance in this respect. Little mention has been made of social values as yet and it seems improper to conclude without giving them the briefest coverage. They are of interest because they are an important element in the broader social context in which disabled people must live, as opposed to the immediate contexts examined in earlier chapters. Clearly, people with disabilities are bound to be disadvantaged in a competitive society which values independence and physical and intellectual skills and rewards the economically productive. Insofar as welfare provision is based on a philosophy akin to those values it must, of necessity, be subject to limitations. The principle that those who do not or cannot work should be less highly rewarded than those within the labour force means that the elderly and the unemployed disabled are destined to remain in poverty (Walker 1980). Similarly, those unable to be economically productive are denied the employment and rehabilitation services enjoyed by the more able bodied. They are thereby excluded from work and the many benefits it brings. Subsidizing employers to take on a person whose work performance is erratic and non-profitable may not make good sense in economic terms, although much would be gained by individuals who otherwise have no way of meaningfully occupying their time or contributing to the common good. While there has always been a humanitarian aim underlying welfare provision, economic rationality has been paramount in determining its shape and character (Topliss 1975). Yet there is nothing inevitable about those values. One organization offering care to people with mental handicaps views their need for help positively; it offers the more able the opportunity to share with others the skills and capacities with which they have been blessed. In this way, so-called dependency is transformed into a reciprocal relationship in which both benefit in giving and taking.

While welfare provision has the potential for redressing some of the disadvantage arising from chronic illness, there are, perhaps, some types of deprivation less amenable to intervention by conventional types of service. While an adequate income, independence in daily living, and easy access to opportunities in the community would help disabled people to maintain the structure of their social relationships, there are likely to be other factors at work which are of equal significance. As Bury (1982) has suggested, we know little about the tolerance of families, friends, and colleagues and how they vary between social groups and settings. We know little about the development of social isolation and the fragmentation of networks following the onset of illness and little of the ways in which individuals might be assisted in retaining old or creating new social support systems. Berkman (1981), reviewing the evidence linking health and social support, has suggested that a variety of strategies may be necessary in order to modify the particular social or psychological mechanisms at work in the individual case. It may be possible to identify ways of helping families to contain or manage conflict and to help members adapt to new roles and responsibilities, and it may be possible to remove the handicap experienced by the non-disabled when faced with a person who needs special consideration. In this way, the lot of chronically ill people and their families can be improved, even within the framework of a system of formal provision which is far from ideal. It is for this reason that we need to know more about the dynamics and nature of handicap than is presented here and to flesh out the bare bones of the model offered by Wood (1980). While this book is primarily concerned with a detailed description of the consequences of chronic illness, it is also intended to make a small contribution to that enterprise.

References

Bayley, M. (1973) *Mental Handicap and Community Care*. London: Routledge and Kegan Paul.

Becker, H. (1963) *The Outsiders: Studies in the Sociology of Deviance*. New York: Free Press.

Berkman, L. (1981) Physical health and the social environment. In L. Eisenberg and A. Kleinman (eds) *The Relevance of Social Science to Medicine*. Dordrecht: Reidel and Co.

Birenbaum, A. (1970) On managing a courtesy stigma. *Journal of Health and Social Behavior* 11: 196–206.

Blaxter, M. (1976) *The Meaning of Disability*. London: Heinemann.

Bloor, M. J. and Horobin, G. W. (1975) Conflict and conflict resolutions in doctor-patient interactions. In C. Cox and A. Mead (eds) *A Sociology of Medical Practice*. London: Collier-MacMillan.

Bristow, A. (1981) *Crossroads Care Attendant Schemes*. Rugby: Association of Crossroads Care Attendant Schemes.

Brown, G. and Harris, T. (1979) *The Social Origins of Depression*. London: Tavistock.

Burton, L. (1975) *The Family Life of Sick Children*. London: Routledge and Kegan Paul.

Bury, M. (1976) Social processes in the development of disability and handicap. Paper presented at Society for Social Medicine Conference, London.

—— (1982) Chronic illness as biographical disruption. *Sociology of Health and Illness* 4: 167–82.

Campling, J. (1981) *Images of Ourselves*. London: Routledge and Kegan Paul.

Cartwright, A. (1964) *Patients and Their Doctors*. London: Routledge and Kegan Paul.

Commarroff, J. (1976) Communicating information about non-fatal illness. *Sociological Review* 24: 269–79.

Coussins, J. (1981) Invalid care allowance, Poverty, No. 48. London: CPAG.

Creer, C. and Wing, J. (1974) *Schizophrenia At Home*. London: National Schizophrenia Fellowship.

Cunningham, D. (1977) Stigma and Social Isolation: Self perceived problems of a group of multiple sclerosis sufferers. Health Services Research Unit, University of Kent, Report No. 27. Unpublished.

Davis, F. (1963) *Passage Through Crisis: Polio Victims and Their Families*. Indianapolis: Bobbs-Merrill.

—— (1964) Deviance disavowal: The management of strained interaction by the visibly handicapped. In H. S. Becker (ed.) *The Other Side*. New York: Free Press.

Dexter, L. (1964) On the politics and sociology of stupidity in our society. In H. S. Becker (ed.) *The Other Side*. New York: Free Press.

Edgerton, R. B. (1967) *The Cloak of Competence: Stigma in the Lives of the Mentally Retarded*. Berkeley: University of California Press.

Fagerhaugh, S. (1973) Getting around with emphysema. *American Journal of Nursing* 73: 94–7.

Freidson, E. (1965) Disability and social deviance. In M. Sussman (ed.) *Sociology and Rehabilitation*. Washington: ASA.

Fross, K. H., Dirks, J. F., Kinsman, R. A., and Jones, N. F. (1980) Functionally determined invalidism in chronic asthma. *Journal of Chronic Diseases* 33: 485–90.

Gallagher, E. (1976) Lines of reconstruction and extension in the Parsonian sociology of illness. *Social Science and Medicine* 10: 207–18.

Gerhardt, U. (1979) The Parsonian paradigm and the identity of medical sociology. *Sociological Review* 27: 229–51.

Glendinning, C. (1981) *Parents and Disabled Children*. London: Routledge and Kegan Paul.

Goffman, E. (1961) *Asylums*. New York: Anchor Books.

—— (1963) *Stigma: Notes on the Management of Spoiled Identity*. Englewood Cliffs, N.J.: Prentice-Hall.

Haber, D. and Smith, R. (1971) Disability and deviance: normative adaptations of role behavior. *American Sociological Review* 36: 87–97.

Hanks, J. R. and Hanks, L. M. (1948) The physically handicapped in certain non-occidental societies. *Journal of Social Issues* 4: 61–7.

Harris, A. I. (1971) *Handicapped and Impaired in Great Britain: Part I*. London: HMSO.

Hilbourne, J. (1973) Disabling the normal: The implications of physical disability for other people. *British Journal of Social Work* 3: 497–504.

Hughes, G. R. (1979) Rheumatoid arthritis. *British Journal of Hospital Medicine* 6: 584–92.

Hyman, M. D. (1975) Social-psychological factors affecting disability among ambulatory patients. *Journal of Chronic Diseases* 28: 199–216.

Hyman, M. (1977) *The Extra Costs of Disabled Living*. London: DIG/National Fund for Research Into Crippling Diseases.

Jefferys, M., Millard, J. B., Hyman, M., and Warren, M. D. (1969) A set of tests for measuring motor impairment in prevalence studies. *Journal of Chronic Diseases* 22: 303–19.

Joyce, C., Caple, G., Manson, M., Reynolds, E., and Matthews, J. (1969) Quantitative study of doctor-patient communication. *Quarterly Journal of Medicine* 38: 179–84.

Kassebaum, G. and Baumann, B. (1960) Dimensions of the sick role in chronic illness. *Journal of Health and Social Behavior* 1: 35–42.

Kitkay, W. (1977) *Understanding Arthritis*. New York: Monarch Press.

Knight, R. and Warren, M. D. (1978) *Physically Disabled People Living at Home: A Study of Numbers and Needs*. London: HMSO.

Litman, T. (1962) The influence of self-conception and life orientation factors in the rehabilitation of the orthopedically disabled. *Journal of Health and Social Behavior* 3: 252–59.

Locker, D. (1981) *Symptoms and Illness: The Cognitive Organization of Disorder*. London: Tavistock.

MacIntosh, J. (1974) Processes of communication, information seeking and control associated with cancer. *Social Science and Medicine* 8: 167–79.

McLean, M. and Jefferys, M. (1974) Disability and deprivation. In D. Wedderburn (ed.) *Poverty and Class Structure*. Cambridge: Cambridge University Press.

Mills, E. (1962) *Living With Mental Illness*. London: Routledge and Kegan Paul.

Moroney, R. (1976) *The Family and the State*. New York: Longman.

Morse, N. G. and Weiss, R. S. (1955) The function and meaning of work and the job. *American Sociological Review* 20: 191–98.

Parsons, T. (1951) *The Social System*. Glencoe, Illinois: Free Press.

Patrick, D., Darby, S., Green, S., Horton, G., Locker, D., and Wiggins, R. D. (1981a) *The Longitudinal Disability Interview Survey: Phase I*. St Thomas' Hospital Medical School, London. Unpublished.

—— (1981b) Screening for disability in the inner city. *Journal of Epidemiology and Community Health* 35: 65–70.

Patrick, D., Charlton, J., Morgan, M., Locker, D., Scrivens, E., Somerville, S., and West, P. (1982) The Longitudinal Disability Interview Survey: Phase II. St Thomas' Hospital Medical School, London. Unpublished.

Pinker, R. and McLean, M. (1974) *Dependency and Welfare*. London: SSRC Report.

Reif, L. (1973) Managing a life with chronic disease. *American Journal of Nursing* 73: 262–65.

Rosillo, G. and Fogel, P. (1970) Correlation of psychologic variables and progress in physical rehabilitation. I: Degree of disability and denial of illness. *Archives of Physical Medicine*, 51: 227–33.

Roth, J. A. (1963) *Timetables*. New York: Bobbs-Merrill.

Sainsbury, S. (1970) Registered as Disabled. Occasional Papers in Social Administration, No. 35. London: G. Bell and Sons.

Sainsbury, S. and Grad de Alarcon, J. (1974) The cost of community care and the burden on the family of treating the mentally ill at home. In D. Lees and S. Shaw (eds) *Impairment, Disability and Handicap*. London: Heinemann.

Scheff, T. (1966) *Being Mentally Ill: A Sociological Theory*. London: Weidenfeld and Nicholson.

Shearer, A. (1981) *Disability: Whose Handicap?* Oxford: Basil Blackwell.

—— (1981a) A Framework for Independent Living. In A. Walker and P. Townsend *Disability in Britain: A Manifesto of Rights*. Oxford: Martin Robertson.

Smith, R. T. and Midanik, L. (1979) The effects of social resources on recovery and perceived sense of control among the disabled. *Sociology of Health and Illness* 2: 48–63.

Somerville, S. (1982) Work and health. In D. Patrick *et al*. *The Longitudinal Disability Interview Survey*. St Thomas' Hospital Medical School, London. Unpublished.

Stevenson, O. and Parsloe, P. (1978) *Social Services Teams: The Practitioner's View*. London: HMSO.

Strauss, A. L. (1975) *Chronic Illness and the Quality of Life*. St Louis: Mosby.

Susset, V., Vobecky, J., and Black, R. (1979) Disability outcome and self assessment of disabled persons. *Archives of Physiological Medical Rehabilitation* 60: 50–6.

Topliss, E. (1979) *Provision for the Disabled*. Oxford and London: Basil Blackwell and Martin Robertson.

Townsend, J. and Heng, L. (1981) The costs of incontinence to families with severely disabled children. *Community Medicine* May 1981: 119–22.

Townsend, P. (1967) *The Disabled in Society*. London: GLAD.

—— (1979) *Poverty in the United Kingdom*. London: Allen Lane.

Voysey, M. (1975) *A Constant Burden: The Reconstitution of Family Life*. London: Routledge and Kegan Paul.

Walker, A. (1980) The social creation of poverty and dependency in old age. *Journal of Social Policy* 9: 172–88.

—— (1981) Disability and Income. In A. Walker and P. Townsend *Disability in Britain: A Manifesto of Rights*. Oxford: Martin Robertson.

West, P. (1982) Disability and income. In D. Patrick *et al*. *The Longitudinal Disability Interview Survey: Phase II*. St Thomas' Hospital Medical School, London. Unpublished.

Wiener, C. (1975) The burden of rheumatoid arthritis: Tolerating the uncertainty. *Social Science and Medicine* 9: 97–104.

Wilkin, D. (1979) *Caring for the Mentally Handicapped Child*. London: Croom Helm.

Wood, P. (1975) *Classification of Impairments and Handicaps*. Geneva: WHO.

—— (1980) The language of disablement: A glossary relating to disease and its consequences. *International Journal of Rehabilitation Medicine* 2: 86–92.

Yarrow, M., Clausen, J., and Robbins, P. (1955) The social meaning of mental illness. *Journal of Social Issues* 11: 33–48.

Name index

The names of the respondents in the survey are to be found in the subject index.

Subject index